Becoming an Exceptional API Leader

Intimate Stories From 15 "Silent Voices" Changemakers

With Foreword by Li-Rong Lilly Cheng, Ph.D., CCC-SLP

www.MaiLingChan.com

Exceptional Publishing MLC

Phoenix, AZ

Acknowledgments

Thank you for accepting all that I am, Cameron, Nick, Alex, and Raegan.

Thank you to my parents, Rosalba and Kan Chan, for the foundations and rich history upon which all my efforts are built.

A very special thank you to my new mentor, friend, and partner in this endeavor, Dr. Li-Rong Lilly Cheng. You rekindled a hope inside of me that took me on a journey to my past and to my future. I am forever grateful for the potential you see in my books and to you for joining me in creating this offering.

I am profoundly thankful to each author for their trust in this journey and for embracing vulnerability to enlighten and inspire our peers and friends. Your willingness to share your individual stories, each so precious, distinct, and cherished, is deeply appreciated. Thank you.

I could never have completed this book without you in my life: Matt Chan, Lori DiBlasi, Laura Stevenson, Patrick G. Poli, Thomas McDowell, and my podcast partner, James Berges.

I am forever grateful to my amazing, international team of experts: Dr. Li-Rong Lilly Cheng, co-lead; Cori Wamsley, final editor; and Christie Mayer, book cover designer. Your support and expertise are essential to the final publication of this book.

Table of Contents

Foreword

Li-Rong Lilly Cheng, Ph.D.

Growing up in Asia Pacific 亞太區 has given me the opportunity to understand the social order and personal responsibilities from an Eastern, collectivist, and interdependent perspective. Being educated in North America has given me the opportunity to be more reflective, independent, and individualistic. The collective culture that I learned from growing up in East Asia is very different from that of North America. The interdependence of Eastern culture and the importance of "face" (the Chinese word *mianzi* (mi-an-ze) 面子, the amount of dignity or prestige that is associated with an individual) have laid a foundation for me and have guided my behaviors, both implicitly and explicitly. "Face" is the attitude that one demonstrates in public, while one's genuine thoughts and feelings are not expressed openly.

Individuals from Asia Pacific bring their multicultural and multilingual experiences to broaden our understanding of diversity. In Penang, Malaysia, for example, you can see mosques, temples, and churches placed within close proximity. This represents the respect for different religions in everyday practices.

The social norms of the East are also deeply rooted in history and trying to figure out a bicultural and multicultural identity is a lifelong journey. Tolerance for individual differences is another area that is worthy of noting, and social obligation is the value that is shared across Asia. As part of their social obligations exemplified by the Confucian value of a duty-bound set of filial obligations— special duties that children have regarding their parents— it is expected that people should privately deal with their own personal problems. There is a common belief that conformity to these cultural rules drives people to fulfill their social obligations, and this social pressure of "face" further increases negative attitudes toward people with disabilities.

But even for those who have lived and worked in Asia for years, interpreting and explaining these nuances to outsiders is next to impossible. This book is about being transparent, vulnerable, and courageous enough to openly expose one's feelings about their personal experiences with people with disabilities and differences. It also attempts to examine deeply why there are negative attitudes toward people who are differently abled and the diverse reactions that the various societies have shown.

There is a general tendency for people from East Asian communities to feel negatively about people with challenges. There is stigma, bias, and discrimination toward various human conditions. In addition, people are likely to avoid having a personal connection with these people because they are concerned about their own "face." Consequently, the lack of personal experience with disabled populations may result in having vague but negative feelings toward these individuals.

These differently-abled individuals have been shamed,

bullied, oppressed, and mistreated. This book features stories from parents who have the burden of shame and guilt and who tried to provide a safe environment for their children to thrive. We are inspired by these accounts.

The process of putting this book together has been transformative. It has forced us to deep dive into our own biases, fear, and insecurity. It has pushed us to open up to identifying our learned values and perspectives which have guided our actions and behaviors. To grow and make change, we must ask these critical questions.

1. What is curable? What is treatable? What is fixable?

2. Where do our biases come from? How can we examine our own biases and do something about them?

3. Is there any influence of cultural values and attitudes toward disability? If so, what are they?

4. Does the social pressure to save face cause delays in early diagnosis and intervention?

5. Should individuals with disabilities feel ashamed? Should their parents feel ashamed?

This book intends to debunk the myth that nonverbal individuals are not expressive, that autistic people do not yearn for connectivity, that deaf persons have no rhythms, that all Asians *kowtow* (act subserviently) to their parents, that .... blame and shame are two sides of the same coin, which needs to be explained further through the stories that are presented in this book.

This book raises the silent voices of the disenfranchised, the oppressed, the invisible, the marginal, the different, the otherness, the misread, the atypical, and the misunderstood. We hear their voices loud and clear. We read their messages as strong and powerful. We hear from the individuals themselves, the parents, the teachers, the speech-language pathologists, the audiologists, and the enablers. We urge the readers to do a deep dive with us and reconstruct your frame of mind. We urge you to embark on a profound journey of self-reflection and paradigm shift.

From reactive to proactive

From disability to ability

From deficit to asset

From negative to positive

From rejection to acceptance

From norms to uniqueness

From treatment to facilitation

From sameness to diversity

From exclusion to inclusion

From indifference to compassion

From empathy to empowerment

From stigma to honor

From disenfranchising to encouraging

From individual to community

From isolation to engagement

From confirmation to advocacy

From invisible to visible

From silent to vocal

From typical to atypical

From prejudice to acknowledgement

Finally, we strive to tell stories and share human experiences that are impactful and inspirational.

Introduction

Mai Ling Chan, M.S., CCC-SLP

Although I have always been told to "never say never," I erroneously introduced my most recent book as the "final book in the *Becoming an Exceptional Leader"* series. With profound respect and a shared vision, I am joined by Dr. Li-Rong Lilly Cheng as co-lead for this anthology, which is dedicated to the intimate and inspirational stories of disability-focused leaders of Asian Pacific Islander (API) heritage.

After reading my previous books, Dr. Cheng, a globally recognized leader and founder of the American Speech-Language-Hearing Association—Asian Pacific Islander Caucus, insisted that I return to publishing with a focus on the intersection of Asian culture and disability perspectives. The prospect of welcoming others into the heart of the rich and storied tapestry of Asian culture—a realm often shrouded in privacy—filled us with an initial surge of excitement. This was a chance to unveil the intricate ways in which this ancient heritage shapes perspectives on disability. As we identified co-authors together and began to receive initial chapter drafts, the profound significance and worth of our joint endeavor became strikingly apparent.

This book, much like the cherished tradition of Chinese dim sum, a meal of a variety of small plates, dumplings, and snacks, offers a "touch of the heart"—a collection of stories that are as varied as they are heartfelt. Each chapter, a delicately wrapped parcel of experience, invites readers to savor the rich diversity of life's flavors. Dim sum, a culinary art form that has transcended its origins to become a global phenomenon, serves as the perfect metaphor for our anthology. It is a "drop of our heart," a sampling of the many different stories and perspectives that make up the Asian disability community—a community we are deeply honored to serve and represent.

Our writers, whose origins span the breadth of America, Asia, and Southeast Asia, bring to the table their unique backgrounds, cultures, languages, and lifestyles. They are the embodiment of diversity, each with their own intersectional identities that contribute to the rich mosaic of this collection. From the bustling cities of India to the greater China regions, through the serene landscapes of Sri Lanka and Japan, and to the shores and heartland of America, their voices come together to form a chorus that speaks of both individual and collective experiences. In their narratives, we find a celebration of diversity that is not only respected but deeply cherished—a diversity that manifests in a symphony of writing styles as varied and complex as the regions they hail from.

The stories within these pages are intimate and revealing. They include the first-hand experience of what it is like to live with autism, expressed through the universal language of art, which allows for the communication of feelings and thoughts that words alone may not capture. We hear from parents who navigate the dual challenges of isolation and prejudice, facing barriers both within their own culture and from the outside world. Their perspectives shed light on the complexities of finding a place of belonging and understanding in a world that often overlooks the nuances of their experiences.

Researchers and scientists share their journeys, drawn to the pressing needs they encountered in the field of communication disorders. Their professional careers are a testament to their dedication to service, to the advancement of knowledge, and to the betterment of lives affected by communication challenges.

Therapists recount their personal stories, sharing intimate accounts of racism, prejudice, self-reflection, growth, and ultimately, leadership and service.

Together they converge on a common theme: the profound and enduring influence of Asian culture, with its rich history and long-standing traditions, alongside Buddhist principles, on their worldview, professional ethos, and understanding of self. Family fidelity, a cornerstone of Asian and Buddhist cultures, is also woven into each narrative. It is the silent strength behind every story, the unspoken duty that compels individuals to honor their families through acts of kindness, respect, and self-sacrifice. This fidelity is not a mere obligation but a sacred bond that shapes identities and destinies. It is this filial piety that sustains individuals as they navigate the complexities of disability and leadership, the moral compass that guides them through challenges and triumphs.

In bringing together these narratives, we find the underlying cultural thread and its emphasis on maintaining "face"—the concept of upholding one's social standing and honor. This cultural imperative often dictates the need for individuals to internalize their struggles, bear their burdens privately, and navigate their challenges in silence.

Dr. Cheng and I each share a personal chapter, and all our narratives together are a study of the power of culture to mold our perceptions of ourselves and our interactions with the world. Through our stories, we take on the responsibility of raising our voices—voices that have been shaped by silence, by the expectations of a culture that often values quiet contemplation over outspoken advocacy.

We willingly and openly share our stories to educate and to ensure that the silence that once defined our experiences becomes a powerful call to action. We advocate for resources, support, and the fundamental human rights of love and acceptance. Our collective message is clear: no one should suffer in silence, and everyone deserves the opportunity to be heard, understood, and embraced for who they are.

In recognizing the academic rigor required of our professors and the challenges related to second-language acquisition in navigating the complexities of cognitive academic language proficiency (CALP), a concept that is crucial for academic success and professional communication within their fields, we honor their contribution to this anthology and we provided editorial support for CALP for academic writing. Their expertise bridges not just linguistic gaps but cultural divides, fostering clinical expertise, understanding, and connection across continents.

In addition, we hold in high esteem the authors who exhibit mastery in their native languages, while also embracing their proficiency in English, along with basic interpersonal communication skills (BICS) that facilitate the essential daily exchanges crucial for fostering connections and community. Preserving the genuine essence of their writing and their authentic voice is essential in bringing their stories to you.

Another interesting aspect has been the intricate process of storytelling and in some instances, translation provided for a few of our co-authors. Varying across a wide spectrum of linguistic and English language experts to a variety of mono-lingual Asian languages, bilingual speakers, and American and Chinese sign language, many supporting family members and professionals have helped to acquire and accurately reflect each person's unique and precious story.

This anthology is a "dim sum" of experiences, a gesture of our collective heart to the disability community and beyond. It is a celebration of the diversity that enriches our lives, a recognition of the challenges that test our resolve, and an acknowledgment of the triumphs that inspire our continued efforts. It is our offering—a "drop of our heart"—to you.

As you turn the pages of this anthology, we invite you to join us on a journey that transcends boundaries and unites us for a common purpose. We hope that these stories will touch your heart as they have touched ours, that they will inspire you to see the beauty in diversity, and that they will motivate you to become an advocate for change. This is our gift to you, a "dim sum" of the heart, served with gratitude and hope for a world that sees, hears, and values every individual.

When Life Throws You Lemons You Make Lemon Lush Pie

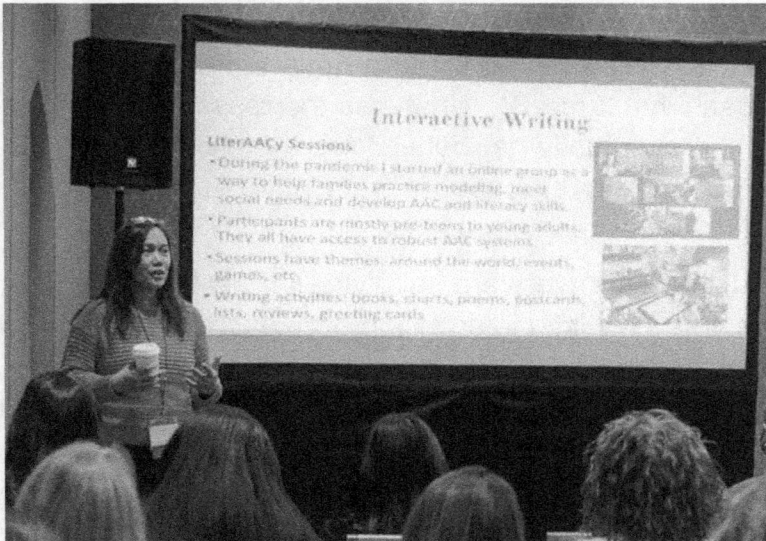

Tina Lorenzana

My daughter Aya was born in 1998. My husband and I were not first-time parents. We already had a nine-year-old son who demonstrated typical growth development and figured this time around it would be a breeze. A walk in the park. A piece of cake. Well, I had to eat those words because those first years were tumultuous.

When I found out that my daughter had a disability, the first thing that came to my mind was "What did I do wrong?" I had so many questions and yet very few answers. I remember when my husband and I first went to see the developmental doctor. Aya was not meeting her milestones. At one year old, she couldn't sit on her own and would just flop forward and lay down. She babbled but spoke no clear words. After testing Aya, the doctor didn't have a definite diagnosis, only that a global developmental delay was present. This was a new term for me, so I had no idea what it meant. What was the reason for the delay? Will she eventually get better? Are there others like her? I had so many questions that were not getting answered. It felt like I was grasping at straws!

At that time we were still living in the Philippines, and there was very little information or support for families with loved ones with disabilities. In 2018, the Development Academy of the Philippines conducted a study, backed by the United Nations International Children's Emergency Fund (UNICEF), on the circumstances of children with disabilities in the Philippines. The study showed that these children continue to experience barriers to accessing basic social services and their challenges are compounded by poverty, lack of data, weak governance, and discriminatory attitudes related to disability in general.

We experienced all of these barriers firsthand. Every doctor's visit, medication, therapy, and surgery were paid for out of our own pocket. There were very few private schools that could accommodate Aya's complex needs. We couldn't send her to public schools because, in a developing country, resources are dire and special education is not exactly a top priority. There was also stigma and discrimination because people did not know any better. When I was younger, I distinctly remember being told not to play with or be around children or people with disabilities because I might catch something from them. I was to avoid them at all costs. Whenever someone's child had a disability, I would hear people gossip and wonder what was wrong with that family. I was taught to value my family's reputation, and because of that, I couldn't help but feel that having a child with a disability would taint ours.

Although Filipinos generally have a positive attitude towards persons with disabilities, there is still so much that needs to be changed (Palad, Yves et al.). In a recent report from the country's Department of Education, data showed that out of the estimated 444,294 children with disabilities (CWDs), only 112,810 were enrolled in 2021. The most plausible reasons for this are discrimination, families' negative outlook on their child's future, and poverty. A 2022 study by the Department of Social Welfare and Development (DSWD) and UNICEF showed that Filipino families raising children with disabilities spend 40 to 80 percent more than those who do not, leaving them with poverty rates that are 50 percent or higher compared to other households (DSWD and UNICEF).

So, after much consideration, we began to plan for a life somewhere where Aya would have the support she needed. We decided to uproot ourselves and leave the life we knew—including family and friends. My son needed to finish his last year in high school, so our family eventually made the difficult decision to split up. Aya and I traveled to the United States, and it broke my heart to leave. My husband decided to stay with my son. His heart broke too because his girls left him. The plan was for both of them to follow after my son graduated, but my husband couldn't stand being apart from us, and we also needed him to be with us. I needed him desperately. After a couple of weeks, he flew to join us. We entrusted our son to a nanny and his grandparents to support him in our absence. Everything went according to plan but then it was my son's turn to fall apart.

I had to go back to be with my son. He needed his mom, and I wanted to be there for him. But that meant I now had to leave Aya with my husband in the United States and I hated our situation. I absolutely hated it. I hated that our family had to be apart again and that we had to leave family and friends because we lived in a country that lacked resources and support for families like ours. It was hard enough to have a child with a disability. It was heart-wrenching to leave her. Throughout those months I was away, she kept asking for me. Aya could not verbalize her feelings, but she had a way of letting us know. Every time her dad would tell me that she would point at my picture wondering where I was or that she would say "Mama," my heart shattered into many pieces. It was the hardest year of my life.

I spent those agonizing months apart studying. I took up further studies in special education. I researched the different therapies that were available. I put all my energy into learning more about Aya's needs and what the future would look like for her. I realized that the only way I could help my family move forward was if I focused on the things

I could do with the resources available at the moment. Eventually, we were able to reunite; however, this didn't mean things got easier. We still had hard lessons to learn. But this time we were doing it together as a family.

When Aya was seven, she was clinically diagnosed with Angelman syndrome (a genetic disorder characterized by developmental delays, speech impairments, and a cheerful demeanor) despite testing negative on the tests that were available then. Even if the diagnosis wasn't definitive, I took it! It gave me direction! I quickly connected with the existing Angelman community, and they were a lifesaver! Apart from the connections I made in the community, it's where I started to learn about augmentative and alternative communication (AAC) and its importance in providing options to aid in communication. I applied the knowledge I acquired at home with Aya. Every step I took was always guided by the question, "How can I help my daughter get better?"

Fast forward to 2019, we decided to have Aya tested again to confirm if she had Angelman syndrome. We did an exhaustive gene sequencing test, and when the results came out, we were shocked! She didn't have Angelman syndrome. She has Mabry syndrome, which is a rare congenital disorder caused by errant genes. As of this writing there are only about fifty individuals all over the world who have Aya's specific gene mutation. You may think we were back to square one, but luckily, we already had years of experience as parents with a child with a disability, so we didn't fall apart. We also found closure.

Then, one year later, COVID happened. Everyone, including our family, went into survival mode. We had to adapt to the new normal. School was online, therapy was done through Zoom, and Aya couldn't see her friends in person. At home, I was the only one who would model using AAC to her. I was worried she would regress in her communication skills. She needed to be among her peers who were AAC users. I realized that other families had the same concerns because they were openly sharing in all the social media groups I was in. My heart went out to them. We were them, and they were us. We were not alone. I had to do something. That "something" turned into starting a virtual group where AAC users and their families could come together twice a week to socialize while using AAC to communicate.

Around that time, literacy was also becoming a big thing in the AAC community. When the book *Comprehensive Literacy for All* by Karen Erickson and David Koppenhaver came out, I dove deep into it. I started applying its principles as I homeschooled Aya. I initially thought that having her learn AAC was good enough. After reading that book, I understood that it wasn't and that AAC and literacy should go hand in hand. I also saw leaps and bounds in Aya's communication and literacy skills. We still have a long way to go, but this gave me so much hope, and I wanted to share that hope with other families. I wanted families to know that all children can learn to read and write, including children with significant disabilities like Aya.

I also took up further studies on assistive technology applications and joined several training webinars and conferences on literacy and AAC. Eventually, I became confident enough to actually teach classes. The virtual groups I started have now morphed into "literAACy" sessions where literacy and AAC come together. At present, I am teaching an hour a day to different groups of AAC users and their families, and it has been absolutely fulfilling in so many ways! I have also started working for Assistiveware, a software company that develops communication apps where I provide support to families, individuals who use AAC, and professionals.

In the past few years I have also presented at different assistive technology conferences such as ATIA, Closing the Gap, AAC in the Cloud, and AAC in the Desert. I love sharing what we do in our classes and I learn so much from the other presenters. At one of these events, an Asian woman approached me after I presented and asked if I was Filipino. She said she didn't remember seeing another Filipino presenter in the past and remarked that I might be the first to do so. Whether that's true or not, I began to notice that I was indeed a minority in the AAC community. I'm hoping this will change, and more Asian Pacific Islanders become more involved in AAC education so that we are seen as valuable sources of knowledge who can bring different perspectives of the disability community.

Aya just turned 25, and it feels like we've been through a lot. Yet, I know there's still so much to learn and do. Some days, I don't have it together; mentally and emotionally, life just gets me. But then, that is part of the journey. And knowing that it is part of it is a lesson in itself. I may not be where I want to be, but I am grateful that I'm not where I used to be. There's a saying that goes, "The best sailors aren't born in smooth waters." This exhilarating journey has taken me and continues to take me out of my comfort zone. It has made me think and rethink my purpose. It has helped me develop a growth mindset, become more resilient, and redefine my meaning of success. Sure, life threw me a whole basket of lemons but I'm making lemon lush pie!

It has also greatly deepened my faith in God which, as a result, has given me the courage to start several ministries, to reach out and comfort others, to teach and share what I have learned. This journey brought me alongside others—moms, women, parents, immigrants, people with disabilities, teachers, and professionals—many who have inspired me and some of whom I've become friends with.

I have also come to understand that my life here is really a sojourn. I am reminded of a scene in the movie *The Lord of the Rings* where Frodo tells Gandalf, "I wish the ring had never come to me. I wish none of this had happened." To which Gandalf replies, "So do all who live to see such times. But that is not for them to decide. All we have to decide is what to do with the time that is given to us." Time is truly a gift, and my prayer is that I'll be able to make the most of it while I'm here on this side of heaven.

My Recommendations

As a parent of a person with a disability, an immigrant, an Asian Pacific Islander (API), a teacher, and the many other roles I have had to take on and continue to do, allow me to share some advice that I hope you will consider when supporting API individuals with disabilities:

- Share your knowledge and gifts far and wide! In this world, where there is much inequality and information is just a click away, be sure to share important resources, tools, and expertise. As the saying goes, "Sharing is caring."

- Don't let culture or language be a barrier to getting services or providing support.

- Connection is key! Get to know their stories and learn from others, especially people with disabilities. Learn from their experiences and their knowledge. The more you know, the better you can do things.

- Work with what you've got. If you wait for the perfect tools and conditions before you work on your goals, you won't get anything done. Progress is never perfect.

- Victor Frankl said, "If we take man as he is, we make him worse, but if we take him as he should be, we make him capable of becoming what he can be." So let's believe—in ourselves and in others. Believe that everyone is capable of so much more. Believe that everyone can be their best.

Change is always hard in the beginning because it's something we're not used to. The important thing is to keep pressing on because, as you keep on keeping on, you find yourself adapting to the change and getting better at it. Just like riding on a plane with a child where you put the oxygen mask on yourself first before putting it on the child, you need to take care of yourself first so you can effectively support the person with a disability. You can't serve water if your cup is empty. Believe me, I know. So be sure to fill your cup continually so you can overflow to the people around you. Poet and civil rights activist Maya Angelou said it best, "As you grow older, you will discover that you have two hands, one for helping yourself, the other for helping others." To do that, all you need is to make love your highest goal.

Ways to Connect with Me

I hope my story has helped you or inspired you in some way. I would love to hear yours and connect with you.

Please feel free to reach out through these channels:

Email: lorenzana.tina@gmail.com

Facebook: @tina.lorenzana

Instagram: @tlorenzana

Facebook pages: LiterAACy Learning Space, Daniel Plan Woman

Facebook group: AAC Chat Group

Tina Lorenzana is the mom of a young adult AAC user. She is an AAC Group Coach who teaches online group literacy classes to AAC users. She also hosts free online hangouts for AAC users and supports families in their AAC journey. Tina has presented in several conferences including AAC in the Cloud, AAC in the Desert, Closing the Gap, and Assistive Technology Industry Association Conference (ATIA). She has a bachelor's degree in medical technology and nursing and a certificate in assistive technology applications from California State University, Northridge.

Works Cited

Palad, Yves et al. "Filipino Attitudes to Disability Scale (Fil-ADS(D)): Factor Structure Validation and an Assessment of Filipino Attitudes." *Scandinavian Journal of Disability Research*, vol. 23, no. 1, 2021, pp. 27-38. *Scandinavian Journal of Disability Research*, https://sjdr.se/articles/10.16993/sjdr.758.

DSWD, and UNICEF. "Cost of Raising Children with Disabilities in the Philippines." *UNICEF*, 2022, https://www.unicef.org/philippines/media/5941/file/Full%20report%20-%20cost%20of%20raising%20children%20with%20disabilities%20in%20the%20Philippines.pdf. Accessed 9 October 2023.

Resources

Angelman Syndrome - https://www.angelman.org/

Augmentative and Alternative Communication - https://www.asha.org/public/speech/disorders/aac/

Global Developmental Delay -
https://mosaicearlyintervention.com.au/global-
developmental-delay/

Mabry Syndrome-
https://medlineplus.gov/genetics/condition/mabry-
syndrome/

All the Way

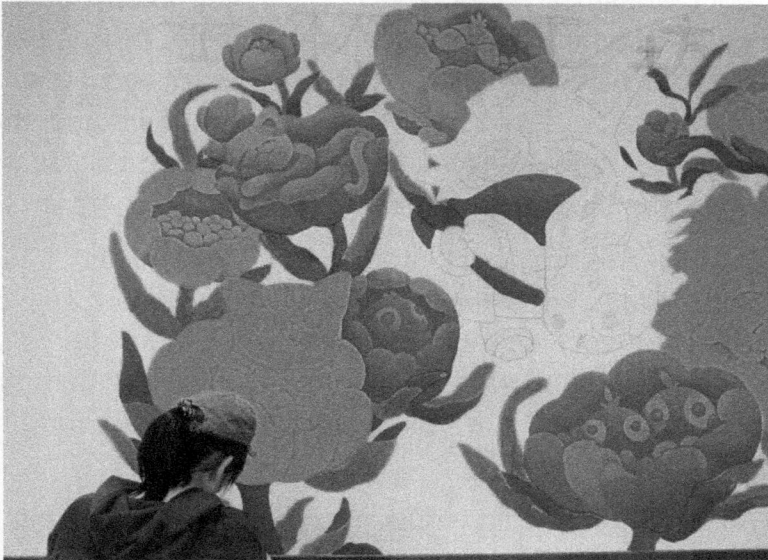

Hua-Hsuan Chung (CookBaron)

鍾華瑄

I know I am different from other students.

When the teacher told a joke and the whole class was laughing, I couldn't figure out why. It would usually take me ten minutes before I could figure out the joke and then I would laugh out loud, which made me strange in the eyes of my classmates. Although I want to behave like the others, it is difficult for me to do so. I practiced laughing, and I tried to laugh when they laughed.

It is exhausting to be different.

When I was 14 years old, I was diagnosed with "anxious autism" by a doctor. For the first time, I realized the difference between me and other people. At that point, I started to hide and avoid contact with anyone because other people bothered me. I could not understand their expressions, tone of voice, and meaning of words, and my misunderstanding caused me to make mistakes.

During a morning study period before class, I was sleeping (sleeping is the way for me to escape) and my teacher was very angry. She called me up and punished me by asking me to stand. She said: "You stand there and don't sit down until you can guarantee that you won't fall asleep again."

An ordinary student would have sat down immediately, but I didn't sit down. I couldn't understand the teacher's real meaning, and I couldn't guarantee that I wouldn't fall asleep again, so I continued to stand, which made the teacher very unhappy. She felt that I was defiant. In fact, I didn't understand what happened during the whole process. It was much, much later that I realized that I might have angered her.

This was the beginning of everything.

Similar misunderstandings emerged endlessly. My mind was going a hundred miles an hour. I was overstimulated, and I had to learn how to calm myself. There were many things that I "couldn't understand" or "couldn't learn" at the moment, but time would be an effective aid. I know that even if it is not perfect, it will get better if I continue to work hard.

At the most serious moment of my emotional disorder, I was anxious and felt trapped in my emotional turmoil. I began using painting to communicate with my inner self. The emotions in my heart could be expressed through the brush. The geometric lines and colors, as well as the forms of jellyfish, cats, and more cats contain my emotions. Painting is another way to express myself and a bridge to connect me with the outside world.

Painting by CookBaron

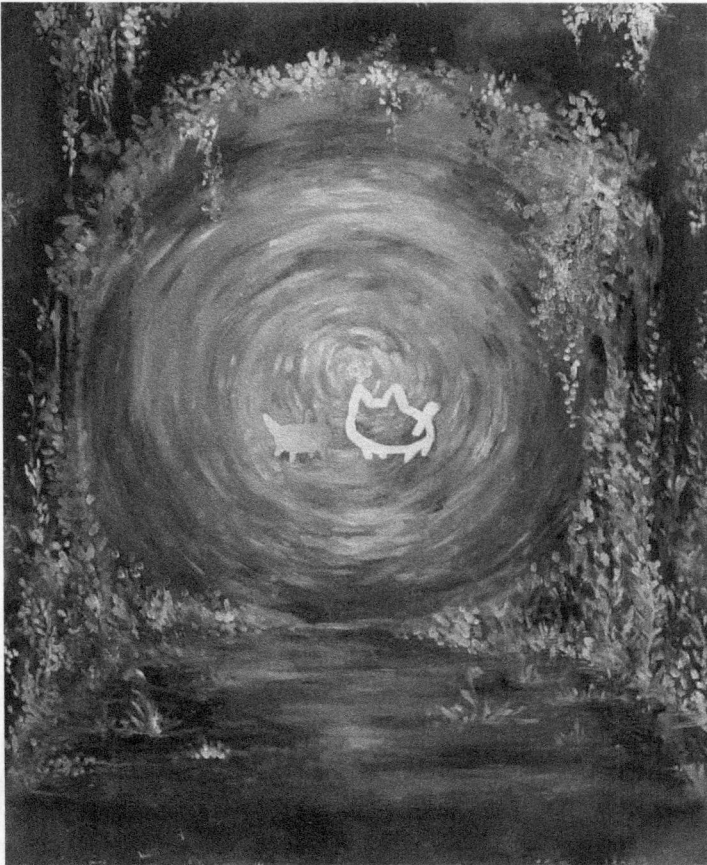

Poem by Mini Keng (Hua-Hsuan's mother)

Looking into the distance

Let's go together!

Scared and trembling

My friend and I,

My friend is bigger and stronger than me, my most trusted
friend!

We move forward together.

I lean on her, I lean on her,

step by step...

Although the distance is far away and the future is
unknown

We still walk together.

Although scared and trembling

We still march forward with courage

===

This is a story of what happened during my freshman
year at Hua Fan University, Taipei.

When I started to compose the picture, I created two
small creatures.

My professor said that the small creatures should not
be kept and asked me to erase them. I complied but added
them back after I got home. I submitted this homework at

the end of the semester and my professor thought the painting was pretty good, but he just did not understand why the two strange little creatures were still there?

I said: One is myself, and the other is my friend.

The smaller creature is myself, and the other is my virtual friend.

My professor asked me to erase the little creatures again. I reluctantly complied again.

Then, as soon as I got home, I painted the little creatures back. I am persistent.

At the end of the semester, I was about to hand over all my work to my professor for grades. I had to erase the two little creatures at home before showing them to my professor. I returned home and I painted the two little creatures back on the canvas again.

I said happily: Great! My professor is never going to see this painting again!

It never occurred to me that my university wanted to use this piece to make cool cards and posters for promotion. Everyone would see this work of mine everywhere.

Painting and Poem by CookBaron

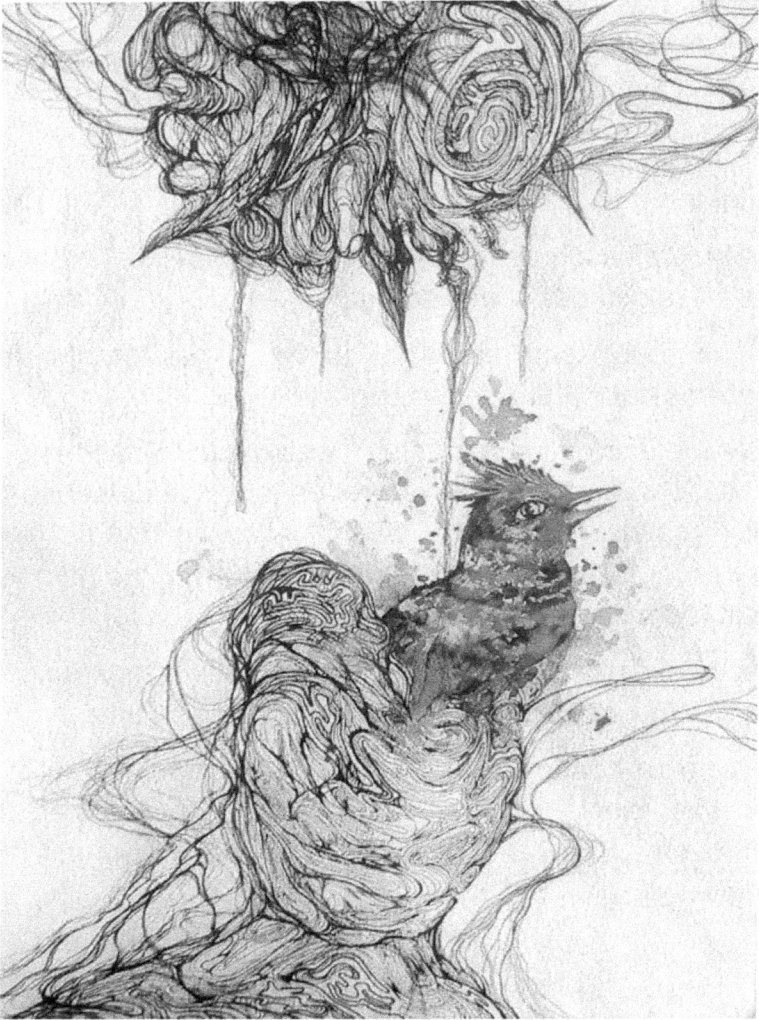

A Voice of Our Own

Like a whale in the deep sea, my scream.

Sounds like a sigh only;

Like a butterfly in the divingbell, my flap.

Sounds like a sigh only;

Like untying knots with one hand.

Each of the words from my heart is unintelligible,

Seemingly calm, I hurry-scurry choose my expressive countenahces;

Seemingly hurry-scurry, I calmy hum my farvoite ballad.

Like murmurs in the pine woods, Lighting flashes and thunder rumbles,

Sounds like a sigh only.

2015.07 Hua-Hsuan Chung

我所擁有的聲音 鍾華瑄

像深海中的鯨魚，我的大聲吶喊，

聽來只是一聲嘆息，

像潛水鐘裡的蝴蝶，我用力拍打著翅膀，

聽來只是一聲嘆息，

就像單手解開繩結的困難，

出自內心的每一字句，都神秘難懂，

看似平靜的我，卻慌亂的揀選可以傳達的表情，

看似慌亂的我，卻平靜的哼唱自己喜歡的詩歌，

閃電雷鳴，松林低語

聽來只是一聲嘆息

~A Voice of Our Own~

How to find a little coolness in the heat?

How to find a ray of sunshine in the dark?

How to find a path in the chaos?

How to hear birds sing in thunder?

Listen with your heart, listen with your heart,

Hearing the voice I have with my heart...

In 2015, I had just come back from Europe after participating in the World Conference on Gifted Education, when I received a notice from the Autism Association in Phoenix, AZ, USA, inviting me to participate in a painting competition. The theme was "A voice of our own." I entered the competition with this picture of the bird above and won second place! In the same year with the painting, I won two awards: first place in new poems and second place in pictures.

Champion of New Poetry Contest in Phoenix, USA

Runner-up in Phoenix Drawing Competition, USA

Painting by CookBaron

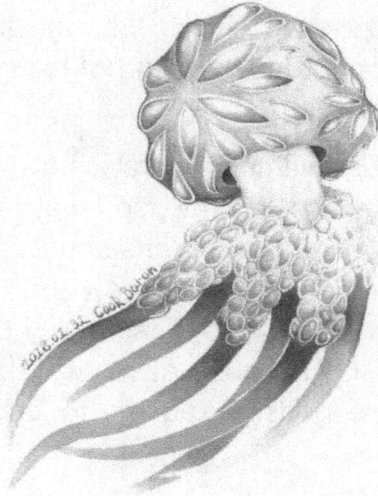

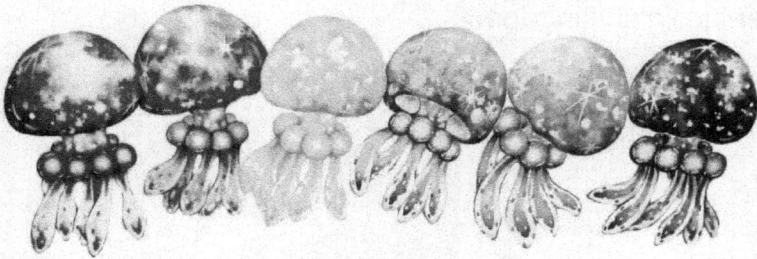

2o2o.10.04. CookBaron.

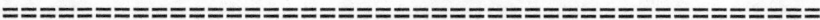

==

In 2017, I suddenly started the creation of Jewel Jellyfish.

Maybe I had conceived it for a long time, and I tried to draw both extremely hard (gems) and extremely soft (jellyfish). I wondered what kind of feeling the combination of the two would have.

At first, I just wanted to draw, but I was not sure how many pictures I should draw, so I went to ask the gods for instructions. *How many pictures should I draw? 10 sheets?* The gods didn't agree, so I threw the bamboo again and asked: *50?* The gods also disagreed. I didn't expect to ask "100," but I did. The gods gave me 3 Holy Whistles in a row! Wow! The gods asked me to draw 100 pictures of jewel jellyfish!

Since then, I have been working hard to draw jellyfish of all kinds, big and small, colorful and eye-catching! My mind is full of imagination, and I will continue to create and draw. I look forward to the early completion of the 100-sheet jellyfish kingdom!

My agreement with the gods will definitely be fulfilled.

100 images of jellyfish will be amazing.

Painting and Poem by CookBaron

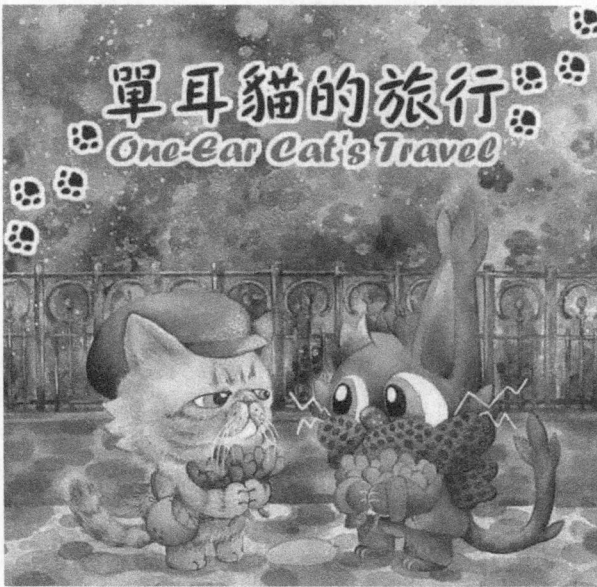

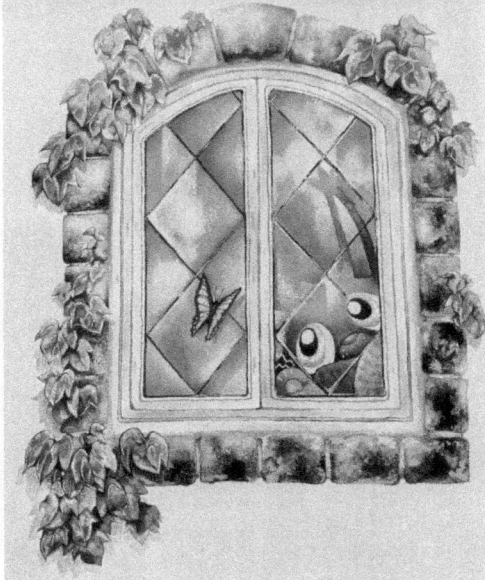

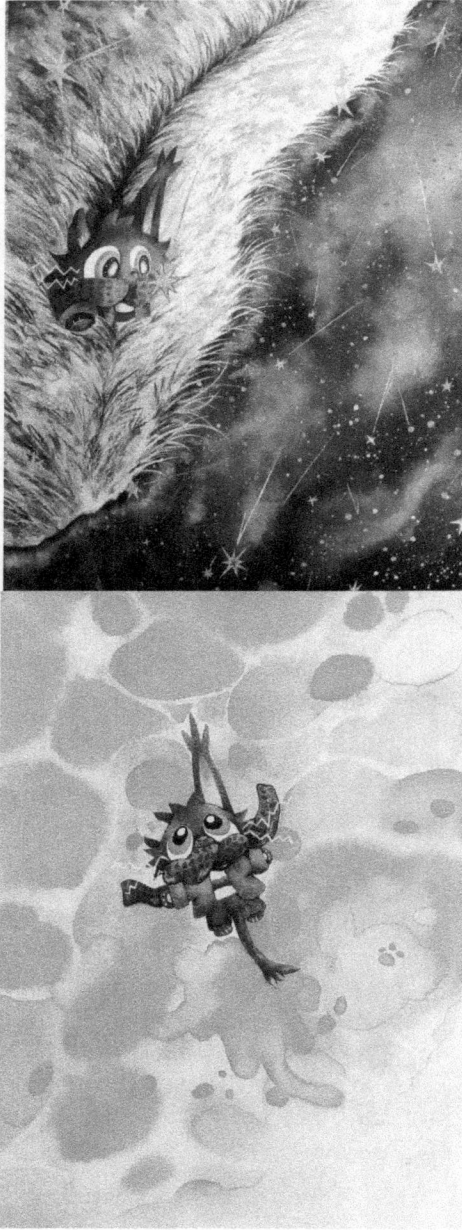

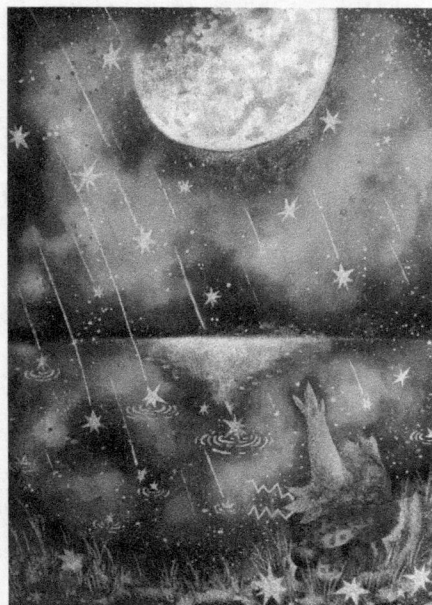

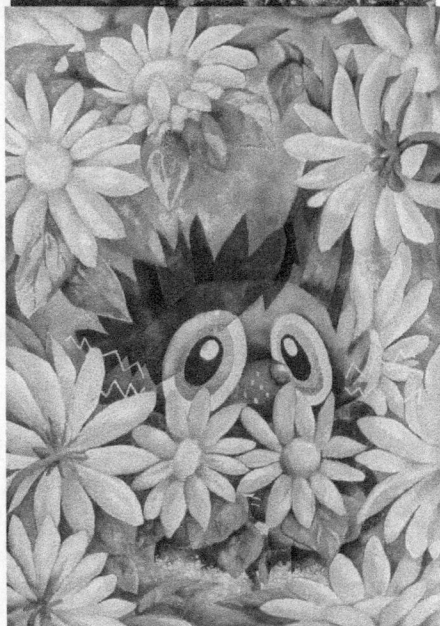

One-eared cat is actually a lonely kitten,

Traveling the incredible world by herself

Learning to get along with life and making new friends

Describing bits and pieces of scenery on the journey

Experiencing the warmth and sadness, surprise and disappointment of growing up,

Still trying to smile and live.

Do the best to bring warmth to others,

At the same time, it also makes herself more comfortable and better.

===

The story of drawing a cat with one ear.

I have been painting one-eared cats for some time, and the thoughts in my heart are slowly presented through the brush: A stray cat travels everywhere; there are clouds, wind, sun, stars, flowers, butterflies, streams, the sea, soft pillows and beds, and dreams that they don't want to wake from …

There is also a real friend for the cat (Han Ji)!

I am the cat, and I roam around freely, but still I have an attachment in my heart, and I also want to have a warm and safe corner!

The imagination is rich and beautiful, and I use various media to express my feelings.

It's really amazing to outline all kinds of things in the

world one stroke at a time!

The more I learn and understand about autism, the more grateful I am.

Fortunately, I have a paintbrush. I use the paintbrush to talk to myself and others. This allows others to understand me better.

I think this is the first gift God gave me.

I am grateful to my parents. They accepted my emotions, tolerated my behavior, waited for me patiently, and slowly helped me to walk out of my pain during my darkest time. They tried to understand my interests and abilities and supported me,

This is the second gift from God to me.

Of course, during the process of schooling, I received guidance and teaching from my teachers in high school and college, which made me feel calm and gain knowledge and ability. There are many unforgettable stories. However, I became who I am, and my teachers contributed a lot to my success.

In fact, I am not a person who is good at making friends, but I was very lucky. I met a few like-minded friends in high school. They shared my troubles, increased my happiness, and kept me from feeling lonely and panicky.

When I was in college, I participated in various domestic and foreign competitions, exhibitions, and meetings. In the past, I could only briefly answer other people's questions, but now I can talk and share with people more freely. This is the opportunity to practice getting along with people that my paintings have given me. I overcame my fear step by step, and I no longer ran away from the crowd.

After graduating from university, I devoted myself to teaching painting to people with disabilities and seniors. After a few years, although I didn't like being a teacher very much (personality traits), I still gained a lot. I can use my own skills in teaching students to create, so they can share the joy of painting. For a long time, I have drawn what I loved. I will continue to move forward without changing my original intention.

My Recommendations

1. If it is possible to keep a pet, one is fine, it is actually very cute, and it will be a good companion and support in your life.
2. Try to enrich your knowledge and abilities and find ways to support yourself. This will give you confidence and a sense of accomplishment and will not become a burden to others.
3. And by maintaining your own financial security, your interests and dreams can be maintained. This is also the goal I am currently working on.
4. I never thought I was a genius, but I worked hard to be a real "person"!

Ways to Connect with Me

Facebook: @cookbaron

Instagram: @cookbaron

Twitter: @Cookbaron07

My name is Zhong Hua-Hsuan, and I am a painting teacher at the Autism Foundation of the Republic of China. Since I was a child, I have suffered a lot because of my poor academic performance. I had difficulty with my studies. But painting is different. I love painting. I have also gained a lot of confidence and growth by painting. Apart from painting, I don't seem to be very good at doing anything! I think that if my work can be seen and appreciated, that would be the happiest thing for me!

Writing Support

Hua-Hsuan's mother (Keng) helped to create and translate the poems that accompany the images.

Dr. Li-Rong Lilly Cheng supported Hua-Hsuan/CookBaron to express thoughts in response to prompt questions and provided English translation for stories initially provided orally in Mandarin. Every attempt has been made to preserve CookBaron's natural communication style including length of utterance, grammar, and emotion. Hua-Hsuan/CookBaron was diagnosed with autism as a teenager. Her mother embraced her and facilitated her success as an artist and poet.

Resources

Autism Spectrum Disorder -
https://www.asha.org/public/speech/disorders/autism/

Advocating for Chinese-Speaking People with Aphasia

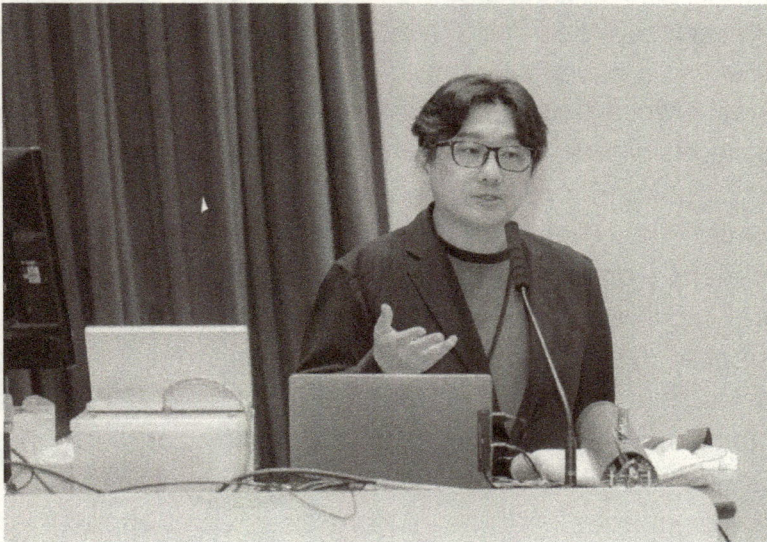

Anthony Pak-Hin Kong, Ph.D., ASHA Fellow

江柏軒

My clinical and research career began two decades ago, after completing a bachelor's degree in speech and hearing sciences at The University of Hong Kong. Back then, the lack of quality aphasia services for Chinese speakers was a complex issue that was influenced by linguistic, cultural, and research-related factors. Aphasia is a neurological disorder affecting a person's ability to communicate, including speaking, understanding spoken language, reading, and writing. It results from damage to the language-processing areas of the brain, commonly caused by stroke, traumatic brain injury, or brain tumors.

Due to the unique linguistic features of the Chinese language, aphasia can manifest differently in Chinese speakers (i.e., affect language processing in different ways) (Packard 1993). Specifically, Chinese is a tonal language, where the meaning of a word depends on its pitch; it uses logographic characters, rather than individual sounds in the case of English, which is alphabetic, to represent words or phrases. Additionally, Chinese has a more flexible word order than English, and this can influence the manifestation of aphasia in sentence construction. Chinese people with aphasia (PWA) may exhibit different patterns of grammatical errors compared to English speakers, reflecting the distinct syntactic rules in both languages. These differences can impact how aphasia affects communication in Chinese and the corresponding strategies used in speech-language therapy and rehabilitation (Kong 2011).

Research in Chinese aphasia has focused on understanding the unique linguistic features of the language and how they impact the manifestation and recovery of aphasia, e.g., exploring tonal processing, grammatical errors, syntactic structures, or logographic writing systems in Chinese. Additionally, research has been conducted to determine the relationship between neural activity and tonal processing or character recognition in Chinese, or to evaluate the effectiveness of various rehabilitation approaches, including behavioral treatment (e.g., Law et al 2006), computer-based training (e.g., Kong et al 2017), and constraint-induced aphasia therapy (e.g., Xie et al 2014) in improving language skills and functional communication in Chinese speakers with aphasia (see review by Kong 2017, Yu 2017).

Critically, the field of Chinese aphasiology is relatively young compared to the extensive literature on English aphasiology. However, the growing body of research on Chinese aphasia has provided valuable insights into the unique linguistic features of the language and their impact on aphasia manifestation and recovery. This research has not only contributed to the development of tailored assessment and intervention approaches for Chinese PWA but has also enriched our understanding of the neurobiological basis of language processing in general.

Several factors contributed to the lack of quality aphasia services for Cantonese speakers in Hong Kong, compared to those in the Western world. One of the main reasons was (and still is) the sheer number of dialects and variations of the Chinese language. Mandarin, Cantonese, and other regional dialects are spoken by millions of people worldwide, and each has its own unique features and nuances. This makes it challenging for speech-language therapists (SLT) and other professionals to develop standardized treatment approaches that can be applied across all Chinese PWA.

Another factor was the stigma surrounding mental health and communication disorders in Chinese culture. Many Chinese people did not feel comfortable (or in worse case, felt ashamed or embarrassed) to seek help for aphasia, as it was often seen as a weakness or personal failure. This could lead to delays in seeking treatment and a lack of awareness about available services. Additionally, the lack of clinical research on aphasia in Chinese speakers two decades ago critically contributed to the limited understanding of the disorder and its treatment options. As a result, there was a significant gap in the literature regarding the effectiveness of different treatment approaches for Chinese speakers with aphasia, and this limited the ability of clinicians and researchers to develop evidence-based practices.

When I was still a student clinician, I was lucky to be mentored and positively influenced by many professors. Their guidance and expertise helped me develop the skills and knowledge I needed to become a successful SLT. My first in-person contact with PWA happened in my clinical practicums, supervised by Drs. Man-Tak Leung and Lorinda Kwan-Chen. They were instrumental in teaching me about the importance of building relationships with my clients and their families. They emphasized the need to listen to their concerns and to involve them in the speech-language therapy process; at the same time, I was moved emotionally to feel more deeply connected to my clients and their families. By challenging me to think critically about the therapy techniques I was using, they helped me refine my clinical reasoning and skills. More importantly, they encouraged me to stay up to date with the latest research in the field and to be open to new ideas and intervention approaches.

This mindset has helped me become a more effective clinician and provide the best possible care for my clients. It was my clinical exposure to different PWA that made me realize how limited we were in conducting Chinese (or Cantonese, in particular) aphasia evaluation and therapy due to the tremendous lack of culturally and linguistically sensitive clinical materials. My initial idea of applying to graduate school and conducting aphasia research was triggered by these thoughts.

I am incredibly grateful for the guidance and support of my Ph.D. dissertation supervisor, Prof. Sam-Po Law, who is an expert in cognitive neuropsychology, neuroscience, and Chinese language. Her passion for research around Chinese language disorders, lexical and sentence processing deficits, and aphasia rehabilitation has inspired me to pursue a research career. Under her mentorship, I completed an undergraduate thesis on piloting the Cantonese version of the Linguistic Communication Measure (CLCM; https://hub.hku.hk/handle/10722/56277) and subsequently a doctorate dissertation on the fully validated CLCM for evaluating aphasic narrative production (https://hub.hku.hk/handle/10722/52723).

These theses represented the very first standardized assessment battery for oral discourse in Chinese and have laid important foundations to additional investigations of disordered spoken output. I am indebted to her dedication, knowledge, and unwavering support, which have been instrumental in my growth and success as an academic in aphasiology.

I would like to take this opportunity to convey my heartfelt appreciation to all of my mentors who dedicated their time and effort to guide me throughout my university journey. Their unwavering commitment to healthcare education was truly inspiring and has had a lasting impact on me. Their encouragement and support played a pivotal role in shaping my skills and knowledge, paving the way for my subsequent success in my research career which, in turn, positively impacted my PWA clients.

My clinical and research interests include stroke-induced aphasia, discourse analyses, development of clinical language/cognitive assessments, multilingual neurogenic communication disorders, and community support to PWA and their significant others. As this core work has progressed, my line of research has expanded to examine gesture production and multi-modal communication in aphasia, neuromodulation and technology-based training for acquired communication disorders, and acoustic properties of an automatic speech assessment for disordered speech.

Since the 2000s, I have actively pursued research projects and knowledge exchange initiatives with a primary goal to benefit Chinese speakers with acquired communication disorders (e.g., people with stroke, head injury, dementia, or related neurogenic conditions), together with their caregivers, both locally in Hong Kong and in overseas communities. I extend my gratitude to my federal funders from the United States (e.g., National

Institutes of Health [NIH]), Hong Kong (e.g., Research Grants Council or Food and Health Bureau of Hong Kong SAR Government), mainland China (e.g., National Natural Science Foundation of China), and private foundations (e.g., Simon K.Y. Lee Foundation), for their generous support of my research projects focused on Chinese aphasiology.

The Cantonese AphasiaBank (https://speech.edu.hku.hk/caphbank/search/) is funded by NIH and is the first language database for studying stroke-induced aphasia in Cantonese. This database represents years of linguistic, gestural, and prosodic data collection and analyses from healthy speakers of Cantonese as well as participants with language deficits after left-hemisphere stroke. It contributes to the field of Chinese aphasiology and informs our understanding of aphasia in a multicultural world. Available for public access since 2015, it has provided researchers, university educators, and scholars with behavioral data from common language tasks performed by Cantonese PWA and healthy controls.

Chinese spoken discourse is essential to comprehend the complex linguistic and cultural aspects of Chinese processing. It provides valuable insights into the language's unique structure, sound, and meaning, facilitating accurate language assessment and effective communication. It also aids in the understanding of the cultural and social context of Chinese discourse, enabling cross-cultural communication.

Given the obvious distinctions between Chinese and Indo-European languages, there is still much to learn about how the Chinese language system breaks down in aphasia. Over the years, I have taken a broad and functional approach in pursuing research work devoted to a better understanding of discourse deficits, linguistic impairments, and cognitive problems in Chinese PWA. These sustained efforts have bridged knowledge gaps of Chinese aphasiology, and have resulted in various types of scholarly products, including refereed publications, textbooks[1], clinical handbooks[2], and linguistically and culturally sensitive assessment tools of language and cognitive deficits in Chinese[3].

I strongly believe that knowledge exchange activities are of equal scientific and clinical values. Through knowledge exchange, we can bring together academic (research) personnel, users of research, and wider groups and communities to increase the impact of research. This process not only encourages the sharing of ideas, data, experience, and expertise, but also facilitates the mutual benefits to all stakeholders involved. Furthermore, an important outcome is that awareness of aphasia can be fostered, and understanding (or empathy) between different communities can be promoted. Throughout the years, I have taken pleasure in providing a diverse range of consultancy services to both local organizations (e.g., Hong Kong Society for Rehabilitation, Hong Kong Stroke Association, or Hong Kong Hospital Authority) and international agencies (e.g., Aphasia United, Voices of Hope for Aphasia, or Project "BRIDGE": Building-Research-Initiatives-by-Developing-Group-Effort).

In 2012, the exhibition titled "Brain and Cognition" was co-organized by the Hong Kong Science Museum and

Hong Kong Brain Foundation. This exhibition marked a significant milestone as it was the first-ever public science exhibition in Hong Kong to feature an aphasia exhibit. It was a great honor for me to be a part of the organizing team and contribute exhibition contents. Moreover, the event was complemented by a "Popular Science Lecture" on the topic of "Aphasia and Treatment," which I had the privilege of delivering.

In fall of 2021, amidst the COVID pandemic, I returned to The University of Hong Kong (HKU) after working for approximately 1.5 decades in the School of Communication Sciences and Disorders at University of Central Florida. Apart from my role as the unit head of the speech-language pathology program at HKU, I am delighted to have had the opportunity to actively participate in numerous exciting teaching and research initiatives, including the development and implementation of the university's Intensive Comprehensive Aphasia Program in Cantonese and simulation of Chinese aphasia in local clinical education.

It has definitely been an exciting and extraordinary journey. Looking back, I am grateful for the invaluable experiences and opportunities that have shaped my career thus far. At present, I am enthusiastic about my current duties, which allow me to make meaningful contributions to the field of speech-language pathology. Moving forward, I am eager to continue my clinical and research work in Chinese aphasia and to further explore innovative ways to advance the field. I will wholeheartedly channel my unwavering passion, dedication, and determination to strive for the utmost positive impact on the lives of individuals affected by aphasia. This will fulfill my ultimate goal to create a profound and meaningful difference in their lives through my efforts.

My Recommendations

As a result of my clinical experiences with Chinese PWA, mentorship to junior faculty members in tertiary education and community SLT, and ongoing education to students in the field, I share some personal recommendations as you consider your contribution to the community of people of Asian Pacific Islander (API) cultures with disabilities:

1. Commit to shaping the next generation of students and healthcare professionals who are passionate about Chinese aphasia;

2. Empower PWA from API cultures to take an active role in their own care and decision-making, e.g., providing education and resources to help individuals and families advocate for themselves and access the services they need;

3. Collaborate with other professionals/ organizations to provide comprehensive and culturally sensitive care, e.g., partnering with community organizations and advocacy groups to ensure that people with disabilities and their families have access to the resources they need;

4. Develop cultural competence to better understand and serve the needs of people from different cultures, e.g., seeking out opportunities for cross-cultural training and education, or being mindful of

cultural differences when providing clinical services;

5. Educate yourself and others about the unique needs and challenges faced by people with disabilities from API cultures, e.g., staying up to date with the latest research, attending conferences and workshops, and sharing knowledge/expertise with colleagues/students.

My Wish for You

Starting this journey to facilitate changes in PWA in Hong Kong and surrounding cities in China and Southeast Asian countries can be overwhelming. Celebrating and acknowledging successes of aphasia services, no matter how small, is essential. If you have been in the field for a while and have some good strategies, consider sharing your own experiences and insights, and offer to help connect them with others who can provide guidance or mentorship. Offering support and encouragement can help those who are starting out on this journey feel empowered and motivated to make a positive impact; similarly, recognizing their achievements and the impact they have made can fuel their motivation and empower them to continue making a difference in Chinese aphasia services.

No matter whether you consider yourself a healthcare professional, researcher, or policymaker, I encourage you to continue to work together and improve the quality of aphasia services, to enhance access to aphasia care, and to develop effective treatment strategies that are tailored to the unique needs of Chinese PWA.

If you are still green and feel that you need more support and inspiration from others, do not feel shy about seeking guidance from experienced professionals who have expertise in working with the Chinese-speaking population of aphasia. Your mentor can provide valuable insights, assistance, and advice on how to navigate challenges and make a meaningful impact on the daily communication and functioning of your clients. Embrace a mindset of lifelong learning, and start different small initiatives by identifying areas where you can make a difference in the immediate surroundings of PWA. This can be through awareness campaigns, volunteering, or advocating for inclusive practices within your educational or workplace settings. Even small actions can have a ripple effect.

Ways to Connect with Me

Email: akong@hku.hk

LinkedIn: linkedin.com/in/anthony-pak-hin-kong-756415206

The Aphasia Research and Therapy (ART) Laboratory at HKU: https://slp-art-lab.edu.hku.hk/

Anthony, a fellow of the American Speech-Language-Hearing Association and Academy of Aphasia, is a world-renowned scholar in aphasiology. His research focusing on aphasia assessment and intervention, discourse analyses, and multilingualism has received continuous funding from the National Institutes of Health, Hong Kong Government, National Natural Science Foundation of China, and multiple international universities/foundations. Trained as a speech-language pathologist, he serves and served as a consultant/advisor to provide research, clinical, and/or professional consultations to many international agencies, such as Aphasia United, the Hong Kong Hospital Authority, and the Hong Kong Society for Rehabilitation. He is also the founding editor-in-chief of Cogent Gerontology (Taylor & Francis).

References

Kong, Anthony. "Aphasia assessment in Chinese speakers." The ASHA Leader, vol. 16,13 (2011):36-38.

Kong, Anthony. "Speech-language services for Chinese-speaking people with aphasia: Considerations for assessment and intervention." SIG 2 Perspectives on Neurophysiology and Neurogenic Speech and Language Disorders, vol. 2,3 (2017):100-109.

Kong, Anthony et al. "Cantonese Apps for Speech Therapy-Adult (CASTA): Development and application to native Cantonese speakers in Hong Kong with stroke-induced aphasia and motor-speech disorders." Frontiers in Human Neuroscience, 2017.

Law, Sam-Po et al. "A study of semantic treatment of three Chinese anomic patients." Neuropsychological Rehabilitation, vol. 16,6 (2006): 601-29.

Packard, Jerome L. A linguistic investigation of aphasic Chinese speech. Kluwer Academic Publishers, 1993.

Xie, Ying et al. "Effect of constraint-induced aphasia therapy on chronic aphasia after stroke." Chinese Journal of Rehabilitation Theory and Practice, vol. 20,11 (2014): 1011-1013.

Yu, Zeng-Zhi et al. "Study on language rehabilitation for aphasia." Chinese Medical Journal, vol. 130,12 (2017): 1491-1497.

Endnotes

1. E.g., Kong, A. (2023). Spoken discourse impairments in the neurogenic populations: A state-of-the art, contemporary approach. Switzerland: Springer International Publishing. [ISBN: 978-3-031-45189-8] or Kong, A. (2022). Analysis of neurogenic disordered discourse production: Theories, assessment and treatment. New York, NY: Routledge. [ISBN: 978-1-032-18482-1]

2. E.g., Kong, A. & Law, S. P. (2019). Cantonese AphasiaBank: Translating research results to everyday management of aphasia 【粵語失語症數據庫】：由研究結果到失語症的日常管理. Hong Kong: The University of Hong Kong (Division of Speech and Hearing Sciences). [ISBN: 978-988-79910-8-3] or Kong, A. (2009). Communication and swallowing impairments after brain injury: Handbook for survivors and family members (腦傷後的溝通及吞嚥問題：言語治療師給患者和家人的指引). Hong Kong: Centre for Communication Disorders (CCD), The University of Hong Kong. [ISBN: 978-988-17240-2-1]

3. E.g., The Main Concept Analysis for oral discourse production (2016; https://www.polyu.edu.hk/cbs/st/en/main-concept-analysis-for-oral-discourse-production), The Hong

Kong version of the Oxford Cognitive Screen (2016; https://doi.org/10.1037/t52498-000), or The Cantonese version of Birmingham Cognitive Screen (2017; https://www.cognitionmatters.org.uk/bcos.php)

Resources

Aphasia - https://www.asha.org/practice-portal/clinical-topics/aphasia/

A Cat Has Nine Lives

Sumalai Maroonroge, Ph.D., CCC-A

สุมาลัย มารุ่งโรจน์

Growing up as the eldest daughter with eight siblings was both rewarding and challenging. My father was an immigrant from China to Thailand around 1932. My father followed his dad to Thailand at the age of seven. He was self-educated and was highly motivated to set up a Chinese bakery store to make moon cakes and cookies from his hometown in Shantou (a coastal city) of Guangdong. He and his father were doing well, as their homemade Chinese mooncakes and cookies not only satisfied the taste of home cooking for many lonely Chinese men who had left their families to find work elsewhere, but also comforted their souls and warmed their hearts. My father was a good businessman; the money he made from his mooncakes and Chinese cookies supported six out of his eight children's education in the United States from 1970–1980.

My mom was born in Thailand to Chinese parents. In traditional Thailand, education was primarily conducted by Buddhist monks at temples, focusing on boys to prepare them for monkhood, thus excluding girls. Girls typically received informal home education on domestic skills and basic literacy. Reforms in the late 19th and early 20th centuries led to the establishment of formal education for girls from elite Thai families, with the first government school opening in 1874. This paved the way for gender-inclusive education; however, less affluent families and those who lived in more remote areas did not have access until much later when the schools were built near their homes. Unfortunately, my mom did not have the opportunity to attend school when she was young due to a mix of national restrictions, family obligations, and work.

Traditional Chinese marriages typically involve a union between the couple and the two families. The marriage was established by pre-arrangement between two families with financial interests as well as social status. My mom had an arranged marriage to my dad when she was 16. She learned how to write simple Chinese, mostly names related to cookies and mooncakes. She helped manage the store while my dad focused on mooncake making. All eight children helped with the store business after school at 3 PM. We attended Baptist kindergarten, elementary, and middle schools that were located within walking distance from our home.

I completed both Chinese and Thai education up to grade 10 and also needed to help my parents with the mooncake business. I was not the best student, but I knew I could study hard and make the grades. Because of the amount of time I needed to help with the store business, I usually missed homework, especially the daily mathematics assignment. It turned out to be a difficult subject of study for me, so attending university was just a dream. As I think back, I consider myself lucky, at least my parents were not forcing me to have an arranged marriage after middle school. Many of my female classmates had arranged marriages and had children before they turned eighteen years of age.

In 1968, I had an interest in learning English, and my parents supported me to study English in England. I lived with an Irish family for 10 months and focused on learning English because I wanted to be either a nurse or an English language teacher. I eventually moved to West Virginia University in Morgantown, West Virginia, and graduated with an English literature degree in three years. I was fortunate to continue my studies in the Communication Science and Disorders program at Michigan State University. I had a difficult time with a few classes, but thanks to several graduate students who included me in their study group, I did well in most courses. However, I faced issues with my clinical supervisor, who would not allow me to do any clinical practicum.

She maintained that the majority of the caseload focused on articulation and language disorders, and because her priority was the patient/client, she wanted clinicians to speak standard English with strong language skills and without an accent. She did not think I met the requirements needed. We finally reached an agreement that, if I enrolled as a client in the clinic for articulation therapy, then the supervisor would provide me with limited clinical service hours. It was a challenge each semester to fight for my right to earn the required clinical hours as I was not speaking "standard English.' I knew the supervisor was using her SLP "golden ear" to assess my articulation and pronunciation of English and refuse my clinical practicum opportunity. I believe that by today's American Speech-Language-Hearing Association (ASHA) standards, her practice would be in violation of the Principle of Ethics IV, Section M.

In 1978, after two years in Taiwan, I decided to return to Thailand due to family obligations and also to contribute to the field in my home country. I was offered a job to work at the very first communication sciences and disorder program in Thailand at Mahidol University. The graduate students were highly motivated to learn and served countless patients at Ramathibodi Hospital in Bangkok. Some of the work was challenging due to limited funding; we did not have communication and science disorder textbooks in the Thai language. Therefore, all the academic materials were in English. In addition, we did not have appropriate instruments to provide services and conduct assessments. Items such as auditory brainstem testings and clinical audiometers were not available. That was when I wished I owned a speech and hearing instrumentation company. Many of the instrument companies had no knowledge related to equipment used in our field.

Even with these issues, it seemed like there was nothing we couldn't achieve together as a group. Life offered us a wide spectrum of choices; we just needed to do our best, be creative, and collaborate as a group.

After facing many challenges and excitement at work in Thailand, I found that I needed to get more training if I wanted to be a competent SLP or audiologist. I decided to go back to school to become an audiologist. I joined the University of Northern Iowa, where I met many helpful professors and fellow students. They helped me understand the complex world of audiology, which is all about helping people hear better. The more I learned, the more I wanted to help people who had trouble hearing. I started working at a local hospital as an audiology technician while still studying. It was tough but very rewarding. Every day, I learned something new from the patients I met. They taught me how important it was to hear and the challenges of having hearing loss. Finally, after a lot of hard work, I graduated. Getting my degree in audiology was a big achievement. It was not just a piece of paper but a ticket to help others. Now, with the knowledge and skills I gained, I was ready to start my journey as an audiologist. It was a simple decision that opened up a whole new world for me, a world filled with the possibility of making a real difference in people's lives.

In 1980, I went back to the University of Tennessee for more study for a doctoral degree in speech and hearing science, while completing my clinical fellowship year (CFY) in audiology. By this time, I was better at clinical work, so the tough courses at the doctoral level were easier for me to handle. All my professors at the University of Tennessee were really good to me. They were kind, helpful, and made learning exciting and fun for me. They helped me get the clinical fellowship year in audiology and found teaching assistant jobs for me with different professors to help pay for my doctoral study. They also helped me get a part-time job at the local hospital to get more hands-on experience and earn some extra money while I was in graduate school.

I also met Drs. Ana and Igor Nabelek, Dr. Defendorf, Dr. Asp, Dr. Burchfield, Dr. Letowski, and Dr. Lipscomb, along with many others who made learning possible for me and helped me stay focused on my goals. They wanted me to graduate with a doctoral degree and pass on the knowledge to my students just like they were doing for me. They were great minds who guided me, and their help made it possible for me to aim to graduate and help students in the future just like they helped me.

I returned to Thailand in 1985, and following in my father's entrepreneurial footsteps, my brother and I created a company to sell hearing instruments, hearing aids, and speech equipment. The business, named "Maroongroge" Company and reflecting the correct spelling of our family name rather than the error on my passport (which remains misspelled to this day), provided a full cycle of service and operated the very first private speech clinic in Thailand.

Our hearing instrument company grew to employ over 120 people, and eventually grew to more than 30 hearing centers around the country.

We represented many companies related to hearing aids and hearing test equipment, speech instruments, and equipment for ear, nose, and throat (ENT) physicians. In addition to making money, we provide many opportunities to help people with hearing loss. Through our clinic, we serve patients with speech and language disorders and represent over 20 different brands of hearing and speech products. Our success was mainly promoting training to the end users, setting up seminars, and training people. We did NOT just sell, but we serviced and operated the business according to my father's advice. He always said, take good care of your customers and employees, and then they will take care of you. Many of our current employees have been with us since 1985, and some retired with good benefits.

Over the years, I have had several life-threatening experiences that have profoundly impacted my life's trajectory. The first brush with death was due to leg cramps preventing me from being able to stay above water during an early morning swim. The second was during a peaceful camping trip at the Smoky Mountain National Park, where a sudden lightning strike severely injured me and unfortunately took the life of the child standing next to me. A terrifying car accident with an 18-wheeler resulted in shock and an inability to communicate, which was written off as me being a foreigner in the police report.

Then arrived the silent predator, a diagnosis of Stage IV breast cancer, where each chemotherapy session was a battle against the silent invader. Covering my head with a scarf to hide my hair loss, I experienced discrimination in the airport while traveling to pay respect to my beloved father in Thailand who had recently passed away. This was followed by a dangerous parking incident where my car slipped into a valley and hung on a tree branch- while I was still in the car! And finally, I feel I lost my life when I was widowed by my husband's untimely death following a brain-stem stroke in February 2019.

Thinking back to my life, I do not feel I lost six lives, but instead, I focus on enjoying every minute of life, doing the best I can to help my students with learning and to focus on graduate schools and completing research projects. I do not have children of my own, but I raised six adopted children, spent time helping multiple countries in Asia developing communication science and disorders training curriculum, and my mission and vision each summer was to bring my students on a Study Abroad Program to visit various training programs in Asia.

Each time I signed my name with the title of Ph.D., CCC-A, I would thank my parents for the degree and the knowledge I have earned due to all my professors at different institutions. I am dedicated to the profession and am currently focused on setting up the Texas A&M International University (TAMIU) graduate program in speech-language pathology. My final goal is to help TAMIU with this mission and vision in the next two years, unless I use up my three other lives! When I retire, I have a major goal to help children with disabilities to communicate the best that they can. There is no limit for any of us, based on my life experience.

My weak point in life is I am afraid to say "No" to all requests, I should be as wise as many of my friends who are successful. BUT this is me, trying my very best every day for the commitment! I believe all things are possible; I just need a little more time to make it work!

My Wish for You

I would like to share a few personal thoughts for individuals who are starting their exciting journey in working with communication sciences and disorder patients in the Asia Pacific region. Nothing is impossible with confidence, perseverance, and courage. Life is full of possibility and opportunity as we take on the journey! Seek collaboration and networking to achieve more!

My Recommendations

As a result of all of my personal experiences, ongoing education, and mentorship in working with communication sciences and disorders, I would like to share my suggestion as you start your journey in working with people or Asian Pacific Islander descent. My thoughts for you would be:

1. You may not become a millionaire from working with people with communication disorders, but you will surely receive more than a million smiles from people who you have given the right to communicate.
2. Dream big, work hard, and never give up on any of our students or patients regardless of their level of

performance, as long as they have motivation to learn. Just remember, we don't meet our students or patients by accident; they are meant to cross our path for a purpose, so serve them well with respect and passion.

3. The field of communication science and disorders in Asia Pacific Regions is both challenging and exciting as you take the journey on the path. Nothing is impossible with confidence, perseverance, and courage. Life is full of possibility and opportunity as we take on the journey! Seek collaboration and networking to achieve more!

Ways to Connect with Me

Email: smaroonroge@gmail.com

Sumalai Maroonroge, Ph.D., CCC-A is an associate professor of communication sciences and disorders (CSD) at Texas A&M International University. She has participated in developing CSD academic and clinical programs in Asia with the long-term goal of promoting an international training curriculum. Her research included speech-language studies of children with hearing loss, Deaf culture, diabetes, dementia, speech analysis, and perception. She participated in a committee for the World Health Organization (WHO) (2004–2008), the ASHA Multicultural Issue Board, the ASHA Board of Ethics, and the ASHA Site Visitors Board. She has been lauded with the Lamar University Best Teacher Merit Award (2007), International Scholar (2013), Global Scholar (2015), and Texas A&M Chancellor's Academy of Teacher Educators (2016).

Finding My Voice to Give Voice to Others

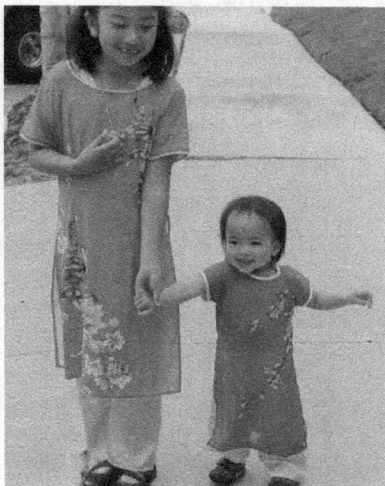

Giang T. Pham, Ph.D., CCC-SLP

Phạm Thùy Giang

My family has a black and white photo of my mother clutching onto me, her baby, both of us drenched from being at sea for five days with little food or water. Our small boat of 99 people was rescued by an Australian Navy ship in 1981. In the picture, a male officer stands behind my mother supporting the full weight of her body. Though her body is flaccid, her eyes penetrate the photo. They are filled with hope and determination.

My mother remembers me as a precocious talker, speaking in full sentences as a toddler in Vietnam. My earliest memories, however, are of me speaking English with my older sister in the United States. We grew up in various small towns in central Illinois where we were often the only Asian or Vietnamese family around. At home, my parents spoke to us in Vietnamese, while we responded in English. Hearing one language and responding in another came naturally to me and my sister. It was not until early adulthood that I switched to speaking Vietnamese with my parents. Only then did I recognize how much closer it felt to use the same language, our mother tongue. However, as a child growing up in central Illinois, I was oblivious to how languages and language barriers can influence communication.

It was during my first trip back to Vietnam that I experienced language barriers personally. As we exited the airport, we were greeted by a crowd of relatives, all talking and laughing at once. Aunts linked their arms around mine, little cousins peered up at me through the crowd. Everyone asked me about the trip and how I was feeling. Even though I understood what they were saying, I could not reply. All I could do was smile.

In Vietnam, I struggled to find words and form sentences. From young to old, people would giggle with delight hearing my monotonous voice attempting to produce Vietnamese tones. Despite these awkward exchanges, I felt love and acceptance. I played with my cousins in the neighborhood where I would have grown up had we not left the country. I wiggled my toes on the beach where we escaped in a fishing boat. My relatives were happy to talk to me and know that I understood them.

This trip made me recognize my parents' daily struggles with language. My mother came to the United States knowing only a handful of English words. I began to wonder how my mother felt when her children spoke to her in English, a language she was in the process of learning. My father, even though he taught English in Vietnam, said he did not understand the spoken language for his entire first year in America. There have been countless times I have witnessed my parents struggle to communicate everyday needs in English, let alone fully express their thoughts and feelings.

More than 20 years later and over a dozen trips to Vietnam, I have reclaimed the language that I lost as a child. My husband and I are passing on this language and culture to our two daughters. With support from my parents and husband, I am grateful that both of our children are able to speak and read Vietnamese. The challenge for us moving forward is to use language for communication. Beyond words alone, our children will need to learn how to use language to navigate two cultures and communicate with individuals of all ages. I want them to develop a strong sense of identity and responsibility to our community.

I carry my own language journey into the profession of speech-language pathology. When I was in college, I had a four-year-old relative in Vietnam with a speech problem so severe that only his parents understood what he was saying. Working with my professors, I analyzed his speech patterns and developed a set of activities to practice the speech sounds he was missing. I traveled to Vietnam and shared the activities with his parents. With daily practice, my relative's speech improved rapidly. He is now a college graduate and a confident speaker.

Learning about the need for speech-language services in Vietnam, I felt that I was in a unique position to give back. As a speech-language pathologist working in school settings, I would return to Vietnam during summer vacation to volunteer with children with special needs and provide workshops for parents and teachers. After each trip, I looked forward to the next one. These trips felt like a drop in the bucket given the substantial needs of the country. Yet it was something I as one person could do that not many others could.

I remember a boy (let's call him "Nam") who had cerebral palsy (a neurological disorder affecting movement and muscle coordination, often caused by brain damage before, during, or shortly after birth) and was about 10 years old. Nam's speech was limited to single words due to his difficulty with controlling his mouth, tongue, and breathing. I worked with his teachers to start a picture-based communication system using laminated photos of people and objects in his school environment. In just a few days, Nam was able to combine multiple pictures to make requests ([give me] + [yellow] + [bead]), make comments ([I] + [see] + [tree]), and greet others ([hello] + [Teacher Giang]). For the first time, Nam had a way to communicate in complete sentences. The joy of seeing Nam express himself made his teachers excited to apply these strategies to help more students.

In working with children, parents, and teachers in Vietnam, I learned how adults place high value on children who show respect. In fact, to be perceived as a good Vietnamese speaker (*nói tiếng Việt giỏi*), children must use specific terms to show respect like *ạ* or *dạ*. For example, I remember a mother commenting to me that her child did not know anything (*không biết gì hết*). When I probed further, she said that her child did not even know how to greet people as they entered the house. To greet someone in Vietnamese, you cannot simply say "hello." Children must refer to themselves and the other person using the correct kinship terms, as in *Con chào cô* [child greet aunt] "I greet you." In Vietnamese, the "I" and "you" in this example change kinship terms based on one's age and relationship with the other person. So if children do not know the correct kinship terms to use, they literally cannot even say "hello." Like my own daughters, Vietnamese children need to know how to use words in social contexts. Our role as professionals and parents is to help children be able to express themselves in ways that adults and the larger society will see and hear them.

Language, communication, culture, and identity continue to play a large role in my current work as a college professor and researcher. What keeps me going is the opportunities to lead and learn from others on my research team, domestic and international collaborators, and local communities.

I direct a research lab of about twenty members. Most are students completing their bachelor's, master's, or PhD degrees in speech-language pathology. We specialize in bilingual development, namely with children in the United

States from Vietnamese- and Spanish-speaking communities. In conjunction with other research teams studying childhood bilingualism, findings from our lab show that:

- Even though children have the capacity to learn two (or more) languages, not all children growing up in bilingual homes end up being bilingual. Children will inevitably learn the language of the larger society, which is English in the United States, because of schooling and community-wide support. However, continued development of the minoritized first language (L1) relies heavily on environmental, social, and familial support.

- There are risks to undervaluing or ignoring children's L1. Language barriers can occur between children who speak mainly English and their parents and grandparents who speak mainly the L1, thus prohibiting the transmission of cultural and familial values, beliefs, and practices. Children who have limited skills in the L1 can become isolated from their own families.

- In the field of speech-language pathology, ignoring the L1 in assessment can lead to misdiagnosis, either under- or over-identifying a language disorder. If a language disorder is undetected (under-identification), children may not receive the support needed to be successful communicators. If a child is mistakenly diagnosed with a disorder (over-identification), this child and their family may suffer from undue stress or stigma.

Current projects in the lab include monolingual children in Vietnam and bilinguals in the United States who speak Vietnamese or Spanish as a home language. We continue to develop assessment tools that will measure language ability and accurately identify language disorders. Our assessment tools utilize children's first language (Vietnamese or Spanish), second language (English), and cognitive processing skills (attention, memory). For Vietnamese children, we aim to support language development when learning a single language (in Vietnam) or in combination with English (in the United States).

My research has led me back to Vietnam on multiple occasions to study language and reading development. Here are some key findings from our research in Vietnam to date:

- Most children in Vietnam are able to read accurately and fluently by the end of first grade, after only one year of formal instruction. This may be due to the high transparency of the language (nearly 1-to-1 sound-letter correspondence) as well as Vietnamese reading instruction that teaches onsets, rimes, and their combinations in a systematic, step-by-step process.

- Kindergarten language skills can predict later reading performance. Specifically, measures of children's rapid naming and phonological awareness in kindergarten strongly predicted reading fluency in first grade. These measures are fairly easy to administer and could be used to screen for children who may need additional support when learning to read.

- Vocabulary plays a large role in reading comprehension early in reading development. Because reading fluency can be established quickly, a focus on vocabulary instruction can provide a strong language foundation that will support reading comprehension.

- Children's attitudes toward reading play a small yet significant role in their reading comprehension. Beyond the nuts and bolts of learning to read, if children enjoy reading, they are likely to read more frequently, which in turn may lead to better comprehension.

Much work still needs to be done in Vietnam to build the field of speech-language pathology and the research base to support clinical practice. Our ongoing work in clinical assessment focuses on how children develop language(s) and how to identify when children have language difficulties. This information will propel future work on developing interventions to support language development.

My own pursuit of higher education was based on a strong sense of responsibility to invest my talents and training back into the community. I aim to mentor the next generation of socially responsible scholars and leaders. I have been fortunate to have amazing mentors who have nourished and encouraged me to find my voice. I recognize how my family and personal history shape how I view the world. These are gifts that I hope to "pay it forward" to others.

Whether you are a parent, student, professional, researcher, or clinician, you are reading this chapter because you want to create change. My wish for you, aspiring change-makers, is to allow yourself to integrate the personal and professional spheres of your life. Often, we consider that being professional means acting or being something or someone different from who we are. In actuality, it is in knowing ourselves and becoming more of ourselves that we can contribute the most to our professions and society. My journey has been the most rewarding when I have applied the following core values to my family life as well as in the workplace:

- Choose to have faith rather than control.

- Allow myself to feel and express emotion.

- Prioritize connection over efficiency.

I want to note that these are process-orientated, aspirational goals. What I mean here is that I do not always reach these goals. I often fail and need to be reminded to live out these values. When I do reach them, I feel the most integrated. The best version of myself. The most joyful. So I will continue to strive toward these goals and persevere.

My Recommendations

To conclude, I share these recommendations for your journey:

- **Decide at which level you would like to make the most impact.** Clinicians are driven by improving the lives of individual clients and families. Educators are driven to support students in classrooms, schools, and local communities. Researchers are driven by contributing to a body of knowledge and pushing the profession forward. Policymakers are driven by building and changing systems at local, state, or national levels. Where do you want to make your mark?

- **Plan for longevity.** Hard work and discipline are the cornerstones of progress. Steady wins the race. To maintain good health, make sure you have a nutritious diet, regular exercise, and enough sleep. Be sure to feed your soul as well—mental health and spiritual reflection are essential. Recognize when you need to take a break and circle back. Surround yourself with people you trust to keep you grounded and help you find your voice.

- **Make comparisons with yourself only.** We as human beings make comparisons. As much as possible, do not compare yourself with others. Instead of looking side to side, look inward and backward. Think of how far you have come. Think of where you would like to go.

Ways to Connect with Me

Faculty profile: https://slhs.sdsu.edu/people/giang-pham/

Research Lab: https://bdc.sdsu.edu/

VietSLP online resources: https://vietslp.sdsu.edu/

Recent synthesis of my research:
https://pubs.asha.org/doi/10.1044/2023_JSLHR-23-00047

Lab Facebook: SDSU Bilingual Development in Context Research Lab

Lab Instagram: @bdcsdsu

Trained as a multilingual speech-language pathologist, Dr. Giang T. Pham works at San Diego State University as a professor of speech, language, and hearing sciences and associate dean for research in the College of Health and Human Services. Dr. Pham directs the Bilingual Development in Context Lab, funded by the National Institutes of Health, to support the development of children with language difficulties who speak Vietnamese in the United States and Vietnam, and for bilinguals in the United States who speak Vietnamese or Spanish at home. Dr. Pham resides in San Diego, CA, with her husband and two daughters.

Resources

Cerebral palsy— https://www.ninds.nih.gov/health-information/disorders/cerebral-palsy

My Journey to Advocacy

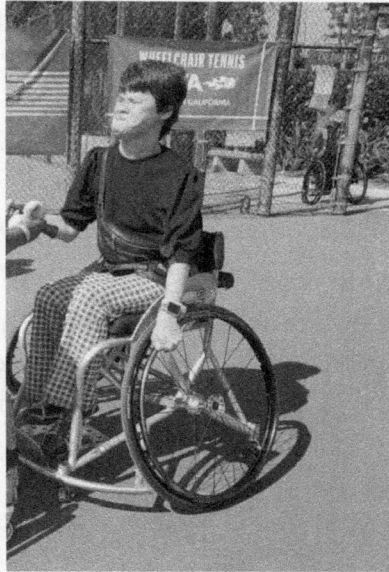

Kimberly Oanh Vuong

My name is Kim Vuong. My birth name was Oanh Kim Vuong. I was born on October 27, 1974, in Vietnam after the Vietnam War. My dad was not with us because he had left Vietnam with a couple of my uncles to escape from the military. My family didn't want any men to go into the service. My dad had to leave us behind, and my mom had to take care of my brother and me.

I was born "normal," but at six months, I had a high fever. There were no hospitals near where I was living so my mom and aunt had to take me to a private hospital. It was on the other side of town, but all the roads were destroyed by the Vietnam War. My mom and aunt had to ride on a motorcycle with a boyfriend of my aunt's. I think that I was in the hospital for a month. Luckily, my great aunt was able to pay the hospital fees, but ultimately, they couldn't get my fever down. That is how I developed cerebral palsy (CP)—a neurological condition, often caused during birth that affects a person's ability to move and maintain balance, as well as their posture.

After I got home, my brother, mom, and I went to live with my dad's parents. It was hard for my mom to take care of my brother and me. We lived out in the country with my grandparents, but my mom did not like it. She moved away with my brother and left me with my grandparents where I remained for five years. After a few years, my dad moved to California and tried to sponsor my brother, mom, and me to join him. However, there was a problem with my immigration paperwork because of my disability. I couldn't emigrate to the United States. without a doctor sponsoring me. My dad had to find a doctor who would take care of me and accept the responsibility. That delayed my coming to the United States. We eventually flew from Vietnam to Thailand while we sorted out the paperwork. As a result, we were stuck in Thailand for almost one year. We finally got my paperwork to allow me to enter the United States in 1980 and arrived at the Los Angeles Airport. After our arrival, we went to Chinatown in Los Angeles, CA, where we stayed with my aunt and dad until they got me into school.

I was only five years old when we came over, but I wasn't walking or sitting up. My CP also caused me to have speech and movement issues. My parents did not know that I had CP until they took me to the Lanterman Regional Center in Los Angeles for a medical evaluation. The Lanterman Regional Center provides evaluation and assessment of disability eligibility and helps plan, access, coordinate, and monitor the services and supports that are needed because of a developmental disability throughout a person's lifespan. I remember the doctor said I would not amount to anything. The doctor who diagnosed me from the Regional Center told my parents that I had mild mental retardation (MMR). I wasn't talking, so I think that is why they diagnosed me with MMR and CP.

I was also crying all the time, and I remember my parents saying that they wished I was dead. One of my parents even tried to drown me. My parents told me that I wouldn't get married or have a career. My parents were never very supportive of me. Luckily, I had amazing occupational and other professional teachers who were very supportive all through my school years. They gave me the right education and assistive equipment. It was very hard at home because my parents were always working, so I didn't get any attention. When my family got invited to family functions, I was not included, so I stayed at home. This went on all through my 18 years. My parents also didn't let me go out with my friends or go to any other functions.

As a child; I went to a special educational class through Los Angeles County throughout K–12. The special education program was in Redondo Beach and Torrance so I was interacting with abled-bodied students. I tried to do my best in school. Even back then I helped with other students to eat and other things. I got average grades throughout my schooling. I received my first augmentative and alternative communication (AAC) device (a tool that aids individuals with speech impairments in expressing themselves) when I was in fourth grade. That was life-saving because people couldn't understand me up until then. I did not care that the device had a male voice. After having my AAC device for a few years my device broke, and my school didn't want to get me another one. I struggled throughout my junior high and high school years. Other students would tease me when I spoke orally in classes. Those were difficult years but I made it. I finally graduated together with 315 students at North Torrance High.

After I graduated from high school, I went to El Camino Community College and eventually moved out of my family home because I had a huge argument with my brother. I went to live with my friend's family for a couple of months until I could find my own place. From 1994–1998, I lived on my own. I was trying to survive. I continued to go to college, working toward my degree.

Thanks to the Westside Regional Center in Culver City, CA, I was also living at a HOME (Home Ownership Made Easy) property, part of the State of California network of public agencies that provide support to the developmentally disabled community. HOME is a 501(c)(3) nonprofit housing corporation. There was a subsidized program for the developmentally disabled community that helped me afford housing through Housing and Urban Development (HUD). HUD paid two-thirds of the rent. It was all based on your income. I was not aware of how to advocate for myself at this time, so it made the application process confusing to me. I had to fill out a lot of paperwork to get into the program, and it was an eye-opening experience.

That was when I became an advocate and joined my first organizational board at Westside Regional Center. Board member selection is based on the following: "The Lanterman Act says that 50% of the regional center Board of Directors must be adults with developmental disabilities and/or family members of an individual with developmental disabilities. All regional center board members are volunteers who want to make sure the regional center does a good job helping people with developmental disabilities."

I was usually a quiet person when I was living with my parents because they didn't understand me. I couldn't speak out for myself. I would never have had life experience if I wasn't on my own. My family didn't think that I would make it on my own. They would not let me go experience things. Living on my own, I started becoming my own person. I met some friends, and I started dating. In 1998, I met my boyfriend through a social group. My friend told me about this group to meet new friends who had disabilities. So I signed up and created a profile to tell a bit about myself.

A couple of years after I wrote my profile, I received a letter from a guy who I had no idea would end up being my best friend and boyfriend. In that letter, he introduced himself to me. Oh, by the way, I still have that letter. It was raining the day we met but he came in the rain, and we had a great time. I knew that my profile would speak to the right person who would love me and make me laugh for 24 years.

I moved in with my boyfriend Brian in 1999 in Orange County. I started working for United Cerebral Palsy and continued with my education at Golden West College. I did not like Golden West, so I transferred to Santa Ana College. While I was working and going to school, I decided to join the Orange County Regional Center (UCP) as a member of their board of directors. After one year of working with UCP, I started looking for a new job. I found another job as a community coordinator with the Dayle McIntosh Center. I was there for a couple of years and organized all of the assistive technology equipment and events. My employment grant eventually ran out so I needed to find another job. However, during that time, I had an AAC evaluation with Orange County Goodwill and became friends with the director of the technology center there. So I called her to ask if I could volunteer and get my foot in the door. I went to Goodwill after my grant was up and was there for almost one year when they finally hired me. I was there from 2001–2009.

In 2011 I earned a degree in women's studies from Santa Ana College and embarked on a career helping other people with disabilities lead fuller lives. For the past nine years, I have worked at the Tichenor Clinic in Long Beach, where I am the co-developer of life skills classes for teenagers with disabilities. I am also a member of the city of Long Beach's Citizen Advisory Commission on Disabilities, where I have advocated for installing beach mats to enable disabled residents to use the city's beaches. I am a 2021 recipient of the Disabled Resources

Center's Jerry Stein Memorial Independent Living Award, which recognizes volunteer and professional achievement and promotes awareness of the achievements of people with disabilities.

At the beginning of this year, I started exploring new careers while still working at Tichenor. I work at the Long Beach Public Health Department as a disability-accessible advocate. I help with emergency preparedness for the disabled community. My job is very interesting. I get to create the emergency preparedness plan, so whenever there is an emergency, I will make sure that resources are accessible for the disabled community. For example, I made sure the disabled community was able to participate in an event for them to get COVID tests or vaccines. I also participate in the community emergency response training, which I thought I would never be able to do because of my disability. But I did it. The training consists of rescuing people. My trainer told me I could do it by laying on my stomach to pull people out of danger.

In my free time, you can find me talking and spending time with my friends. I love to travel and have been to many exciting places. I would love to say that Canada has to be my favorite place. It felt like home to me. I love going to Arizona for spring training to watch the Dodgers play baseball. I love food. I like to try different foods when we travel. Another thing I like to do in my free time is try different sports. I am taking karate right now. One of my favorite sports activities is riding horses. Because I like adaptive sports, I am helping to organize the first adaptive sports fair in the city of Long Beach. I saw there was a need for an adaptive sports program in the city.

My Recommendations

As a result of all of my experiences, ongoing education, and mentorship, I share these personal recommendations with you as you consider your contribution to the community of people of Asian Pacific Islander culture with disabilities: I would recommend to family and professionals who are working with people with disabilities to expect them to make something of themselves and their lives. I also recommend that you don't baby them or try doing everything for them. Give them the education that they deserve. Teach them how to advocate for themselves. Become their biggest advocate.

My Wish for You

People who are Asian can be very quiet and reserved. I would like families to speak up for their children with disabilities. I want to speak honestly: families who have trouble with their children who have disabilities may not know the future potential of their child. They need to know of all the great resources out there for their child and need to learn how to advocate for them.

Ways to Connect with Me

Email: kimvunong1974@gmail.com

LinkedIn: www.linkedin.com/in/kim-vuong-2865777

Facebook: www.facebook.com/kim.vuong.92

Instagram: https://www.instagram.com/kvuong74/

Oanh "Kim" Vuong was born in Vietnam in 1974 and immigrated to the United States in 1980. Since childhood, she has lived with cerebral palsy, a condition that has made it a challenge to do many things that other people take for granted, from walking on the beach to speaking to a group. Nevertheless, she earned a degree in women's studies from Santa Ana College and embarked on a career helping other people with disabilities lead fuller lives. For the past nine years, she's worked at the Tichenor Clinic in Long Beach, where she is the co-developer of life skills classes for teenagers with disabilities. She is also a member of the city of Long Beach's Citizen Advisory Commission on Disabilities, where she advocated for installing beach mats to enable disabled residents to use the city's beaches. She is a 2021 recipient of the Disabled Resources Center's Jerry Stein Memorial Independent Living Award, which recognizes volunteer and professional achievement and promotes awareness of the achievements of people with disabilities.

Finding Self-Love in a Diagnosis

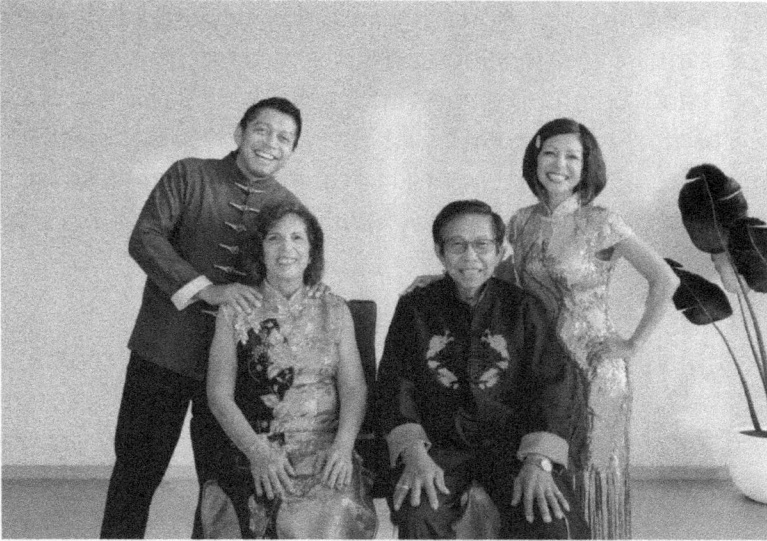

Mai Ling Chan, M.S., CCC-SLP

陳美玲

My next trip isn't for two weeks, but my suitcase is open on the floor, and I have already packed a few outfits, most of my socks, underwear, pajamas, and a few sweatshirts. I have a lengthy checklist accessible on my phone and computer regarding work-related tasks, in addition to another hand-written one on the kitchen counter to cover house-related tasks that need to be completed before I leave. And I have begun a gradual, but intricate system of sorting vitamins and other health items into Ziploc bags so I am sure to have all the essentials readily available.

To an onlooker, the scene would seem like the actions of someone who is highly organized and excited about their upcoming trip. And they wouldn't be wrong. There's a certain thrill I get in planning for a new journey, selecting outfits, and ensuring every necessity has been accounted for. But this routine isn't just born from excitement; it's a strategy, crafted over years, to tackle the emotional strain that intensifies due to the mounting anxiety inherent in preparations left to the eleventh hour.

In retrospect, I acknowledge that my entire childhood was a daily challenge to somehow harness my overactive mind and focus long enough to complete required, mundane, or multi-step tasks. I could easily make any task interesting by adding a component of creativity and play— which typically led to hyperfocus, time blindness (being unaware of the passing time), and ultimately, poor time management for the other things I was supposed to be getting done. Although I was an only child until I was 12 years old, I never felt lonely because of the constant chatter in my brain. I didn't understand it then, but I can now describe the ability to have four to five thoughts occurring simultaneously. This typically includes a song playing on a loop, plus any variety of task management, future planning, random thoughts and questions, favorite people or memories popping into my mind, and... intermittent thoughts of guilt and shame related to missed deadlines, appointments, tasks, goals, etc.

In addition to my buzzing, self-entertaining, multi-topic mental activity, my body also seemed to have a rhythm of its own. Bruises on my shins manifested daily from frequent bumps with furniture and clumsy tumbles, items were constantly misplaced as my hands seemed to function on their own agenda, and glasses of water were in constant peril if they were placed within arm's reach.

Although I was considered "gifted," advancing to first grade during the first half of my kindergarten year, I struggled to perform within the system. Despite my vibrant inner world, while I soared in some areas, I often received a few C's on every report card through 8th grade. I was typically on the teacher's radar for distracting my fellow students, not paying attention or staying on task, and not having my homework assignments. My desk was an absolute mess, and I could never find things I needed. When I went out with my parents, I was often lost in a store because I was playing, daydreaming, or focused on a product. I was always talking too much, demanding attention in almost every situation, and likely considered rude in social situations. In my early years, I was often referred to as having "no filters," as in sharing overtly personal or otherwise private information with disregard for other people's feelings and using sarcasm and humor in hurtful ways. I'd like to blame it on my New Jersey "social culture," but it is more likely that my actions were self-absorbed and egocentric to a fault.

In the 1970s, labels and diagnoses weren't referred to as prominently as they are today. Back then, I was seen as a "chatty girl" with boundless curiosity, energy, and lots of "potential." My parents were well aware of my hyperactivity and flair for the dramatic and relied on their personal cultural upbringings and experiences to help shape me. My mother is Colombian and first-generation American, and my father is Chinese from Hong Kong. He came to America in his early 20s and earned his citizenship by fighting and surviving the Vietnam War. I was born shortly after his return.

Although my father assimilated well into American society over the years, he has always maintained strong ties to Chinese culture and teachings. He dutifully sponsored his parents to become U.S. citizens, and I grew up with both paternal grandparents living in our home. Growing up as one of only two Chinese families in Keyport, a small fishing town in New Jersey, I was immersed in Chinese life, eating traditional family-style meals with a bowl of rice and chopsticks when I was six years old, watching bean sprouts grow magically in a bucket in my grandfather's bedroom, and waiting excitedly for a delivery of fresh *char siu bao* from the bakery in Chinatown, NY.

In an effort to reduce my disordered, clumsy, and verbose lifestyle, my father encouraged focused and constructive thinking. He tried to harness and moderate my "monkey mind"—a term from Buddhist principles that denotes an unsettled, restless, or confused state of mind—by employing public disapproval as a deterrent, aiming to cultivate self-control and a sense of accountability in me. He frequently cautioned, "People are always watching you. Everything you do and don't do. Your actions speak louder than your words. You don't have to say everything you're thinking. Just do the right thing, the BEST thing, and you will be rewarded for your actions. Always do your best work. Never show laziness." And the most impactful, "Everything you do out there represents your family." He also attempted to provide organizational tips, "Don't rush your work. Take your time. Slow it down. Focus on each step, and do them correctly. Pay attention to what you are doing, always."

This sounds like wisdom from Buddha himself. My father's guidance steeped in his Chinese heritage—emphasizing diligence, accountability, and respect—were intended as pillars to ground me and my kaleidoscope mind. But alas, little girls hear and internalize words differently than adults.

My unique cultural background was also a double-edged sword. On one hand, I had the privilege of experiencing the world through a blended lens of Colombian and Chinese heritage. On the other, this duality often clashed with the world outside. During this time I was also privately struggling to exist in the duality of American culture and catholic school regimens mixed with a culturally rich Chinese homelife. Multiple factors contributed to my distinct experience. I was a year younger than my classmates and my cultural background stood out starkly, underscored by my unique name in contrast to the more common Caucasian names like "Jennifer," "Lisa," and "Anne." Additionally, my family was not in the same income level and social circles as my peers, and I held the distinction of being the sole student of Chinese descent in my grammar school classes, even though I'm only half Chinese.

Adding to these cultural differences, my childhood personality was what they now refer to as "extra"—talked too much, tried too hard to win friends over, pushed the envelope with too many sarcastic jokes, demanded too much attention, etc. I was also oblivious to the fact that my clothes weren't in vogue, that my Chinese meals might be considered "unconventional" by my friends who came over for a playdate and stayed for dinner, and that spending weekends engrossed in kung fu movies with my grandparents was quite out of the ordinary. I only knew that I was a sad fifth grader when I wasn't invited to sit in groups at the lunch table or invited to "popular" student's parties. I also recall the mix of confusion and shame during report card time. It was hard enough grappling with my own academic performance, but even harder when a "friend" said racial statements they had learned from their parents such as "I thought Asians were supposed to be good at Math." and "Oh! You aren't as smart as I thought you were cuz you're Chinese." These were my earliest experiences with the unspoken assumptions and expectations related to Asian academic bias.

As a result of my social anxiety, organizational dysfunction, and academic struggles, I gradually developed a veil of shame and guilt related to disappointment and failure. That little girl erroneously misinterpreted well-meant teachings into an unattainable bar of achievement. Sadly, she kept missing the bar, not because of a lack of will or ambition, but because she didn't have the essential skills to plan, prepare, support, and ultimately achieve her goals.

Beginning in high school, I began a series of self-preservation tactics and independently devised intricate systems and processes for the organization and execution of tasks. Driven to shed my previous reputation, I was able to reinvent my outward presentation as a highly organized, effective, and dependable student, but inwardly, I berated myself constantly for minor missteps as I continued to hone my new skills. I knew from my father's teachings that "Everyone is always watching you," and I did not want to slip back into my previous chaos. As you can imagine, this mindset resulted in a lifetime of internal struggle, including constant anxiety, mild obsessive-compulsive tendencies (OCD), and unhealthy relationships.

Thankfully I have effectively "self-managed" and grown exponentially over the years. I am blessed to have supportive and loving family and friends who appreciate my brilliant mind and energy, and accept the whirlwind and organized chaos that is my daily life. As many other neurodivergent individuals agree, I have always referred to my active mind as my personal superpower.

The idea of attention deficit disorder (ADHD) wasn't on my personal radar until recently. During the past two years, I have had the benefit of hearing from friends, and colleagues who have been recently diagnosed with ADHD. As a speech-language pathologist, I have supported several students with ADHD to identify processes and systems to help support their educational goals, and not once did I find commonalities with their needs. But in listening to adult women share their personal journeys I found many relatable themes that made me wonder if I too had ADHD. The symptoms that present in an adult woman are different from those of a young girl. The patterns they described resonated with me, such as a history of anxiety, organizational obsessions, frequent errors when writing or typing, speed reading, not following through on multi-step processes, and difficulty paying attention to details—at times it was like looking into a mirror. I eventually decided to go through the process of formal evaluation.

This process was an important step and felt necessary.

One early morning, I completed a very lengthy and thorough intake questionnaire. The process of recalling and reporting on the details of my chaotic youth was cathartic and informative. Memories came flooding back—memories of embarrassment, feeling out of place, and being overwhelmed—it all came rushing forth. In line with the values of my upbringing, I worked diligently to provide an abundance of information—"Always do your best!"—to ensure that the evaluator had the necessary context to draw an accurate conclusion.

After ensuring I had thoroughly answered every question, I shut my laptop. Emotions overwhelmed me, and tears streamed freely. I knew for sure that I would qualify for the diagnosis, and I suddenly felt like a giant weight had been lifted from my body.

It isn't my fault that I have such an overactive mind.

My struggles are not a result of a lazy mindset.

I am not a disappointment.

I am doing the best I can.

The diagnosis wasn't just a label; it was validation. It reframed my past, provided context, and offered a path forward. Since receiving the final letter from my physician, I have been learning so much more about myself and my beautiful mind. The more I read and talk with other people, the more I am able to identify my self-talk and begin to shift my personal perspective. I now understand the meaning of "masking" (camouflaging symptoms by controlling impulses, rehearsing responses, and copying socially acceptable behaviors) and how I have employed this strategy throughout my life. I am able to identify the frequent anxiety that creeps into my day and create space for simple breathing techniques or full yoga sessions to reduce and sometimes eliminate the feeling completely. I am exploring the benefits and challenges of medication in order to make an informed decision.

I have found connections with several Asian women who have been diagnosed with ADHD and serve as inspirations, sharing their personal journeys, pioneering technologies to aid those with ADHD, and taking on leadership roles within neurodiverse communities. I experience so much joy in sharing their work and offerings through all of my professional channels to help reach more women like myself who may be struggling and haven't recognized the possibility that neurodiversity may be a critical piece of their story. In an attempt to show my deep gratitude to the community, I have also shared my journey on my podcast and on social media and have been contacted by many friends, colleagues, and listeners who found similarities, comparing their lives to my experience, and are beginning their own journeys to make sense of their beautiful minds.

And finally, I am sharing my story with you because I trust the process and value of storytelling.

This story is not just mine. It's the story of countless individuals navigating the intricate maze of neurodiversity. I've heard the dismissive comment, "Everyone claims they have ADHD." I aim to shed light on the deeply personal and emotional path to identifying with this diagnosis, in the hopes of enhancing awareness, erasing stigmas, and fostering empathy and understanding.

My Recommendations

As a result of my personal experiences with disability, as both a professional and an individual, I offer the following as gentle reminders that you are always capable of learning, growing, and becoming the highest form of self-actualization.

1. **Continue to seek knowledge.** You never know when something or someone will profoundly touch your life.

2. **Learn about Self-Love.** Delving into understanding and cherishing oneself can be the cornerstone of an unexpected and memorable journey.

3. **Tune in to your self-talk.** Listening to your inner dialogue can shape how you interpret specific events, fostering a deeper connection to yourself and the world around you.

This is the fourth book in my *Becoming an Exceptional Leader* series, and during the early planning stages for each book, I have consistently paused to consider the value of including a personal chapter. Each time, I have compared my story with the other amazing co-authors' and wondered if it would be as compelling and helpful. Thankfully, you have let me know in your feedback and emails that you resonate with my stories, feel a connection with me, and ultimately enjoy my contribution. With that said, I trust this fresh chapter of my life will provide further insight and deepened connection with me as well as the growing number of Asian women and other adults who are on a journey of self-discovery. And I encourage you to courageously examine your own life journey and those of your friends and families with an open mind and heart. Never stop learning about yourself. You are beautiful.

My Community

Listen to my episode about my journey with ADHD and an interview with Chris Wang, CEO of the Shimmer app on the Xceptional Leaders podcast:

Living with ADHD in Adulthood with Chris Wang
https://bit.ly/ADHD-Mai

Ways to Connect with Me

www.mailingchan.com
Twitter: https://twitter.com/mailingchan
Linked In: https://www.linkedin.com/in/mailingchan
Facebook: https://www.facebook.com/MaiLingChanSLP
Instagram: @mailingchan

Becoming an Exceptional API Leader

Mai Ling is a speech-language pathologist, industry historian, global connector, keynote speaker, and technology entrepreneur. Building on a lifetime of successful ventures, she focuses on supporting disability-focused thought leaders and building a global ecosystem to support innovative and assistive technologies. As an executive consultant, and through Exceptional Lab, she facilitates national and international partnerships with disability experts and supports strategic business development. In addition to supporting the Becoming an Exceptional Series publications, Mai Ling continues to spotlight industry leaders on the Xceptional Leaders podcast, now in its sixth year, reaching listeners in over 140 countries.

For more information about ADHD in adults, visit the Attention Deficit Disorder Association: https://add.org/

Triumph over Challenges:
A Parent's Journey

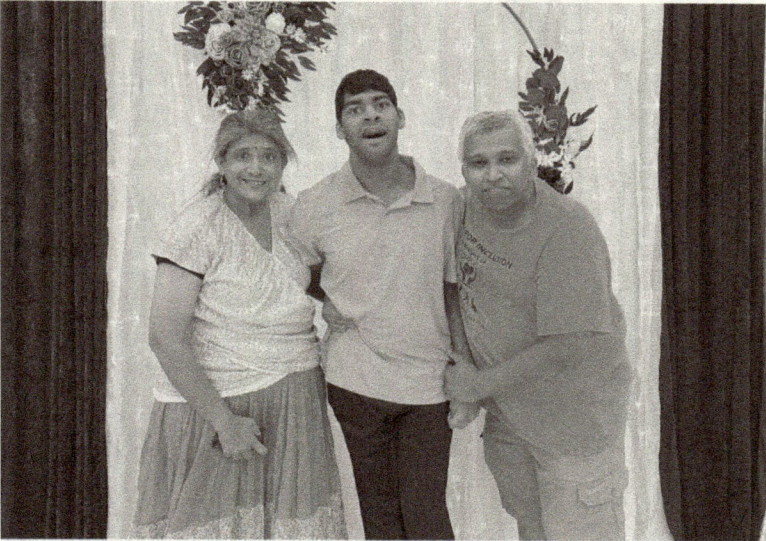

Meena Kalyanasundaram

Challenges in my parenting journey started the day my first child was born and continue until today. My husband and I were first-generation immigrants from India and by the time Athish was born, we had already been living in the United States for more than 25 years. My husband's job was the primary source of income, and we faced the common struggles of immigrants in adjusting to the American culture, food, and the insurance system.

Becoming an Exceptional API Leader

In 1998 I was 30 years old and pregnant. What were supposed to be moments of celebration, turned out to be shock and devastation. I was admitted to the hospital on May 18, 1998, with a low-grade fever and although I had a normal delivery, the happiness of Athish's entry into my life, lasted just a few moments as we noticed that the umbilical cord was rounded five times tightly around the baby's neck and he had no movements. There was no crying. He was like a doll. Newborns are rated on the APGAR scale, a standardized assessment immediately after birth of a newborn's condition, comprised of five components: 1) color, 2) heart rate, 3) reflexes, 4) muscle tone, and 5) respiration, each of which is given a score of 0, 1, or 2. He had a score of zero at one minute, and one at five minutes. Faced with an APGAR score of one, which indicated the newborn was struggling, the team quickly recognized the infant had hypoxic-ischemic encephalopathy (HIE), (caused by lack of oxygen to the brain before or shortly after birth), one of the most severe complications that can affect full-term infants. Hospital staff put him on a ventilator to breathe. While I was eager to hold my newborn, he disappeared, and I was told he was taken to the nursery. Our joy instantly turned to sorrow, confusion, and panic.

While we were waiting to see the baby, we held onto the hopeful thought, "It's a routine thing" until the nurses came back saying that the child was depressed and they were still checking on him. I wasn't able to believe it and didn't take it seriously until they brought him to my bed while hooked up to a ventilator. I touched him with my little pinky, with my tears streaming down onto him, but his hands, legs, and entire body were frozen. I was updated by the nurses again, that he was depressed, and he needed to be on life support. Nurses told me that my newborn was going to be transferred to Stanford Hospital's Neonatal Intensive Care Unit (NICU).

In the days that followed, we didn't know what was really going on, or what would happen to our baby. "Your child is depressed." "Your child's brain is damaged." "We have kept him in the NICU, and it is very difficult for him to survive." When the doctors said this, my family members cried. This grief affected my father and he, being a heart patient, developed a mild cardiac attack and was rushed to his cardiologist. What they said sounded Greek and Latin to my husband and me, and we were so confused and overwhelmed.

But I was in the firm belief that my son would survive.

We had health maintenance organization (HMO) insurance through my husband's job, but without full understanding of how the hospital and insurance works in this country, both me and my husband felt totally lost in a big ocean. We were told that insurance would not be able to cover the hospital stay and that they would stop the treatments. We were told that the baby should be taken out of the ventilator because it would be difficult to claim reimbursement from the insurance. On the fourth day of his life, the physicians said, "We will treat him for one more day and will stop the treatment and give him to you, and he may be able to survive only for a few minutes." When this was uttered, I broke down and wailed. That was the last day I cried for my son.

When they took the baby out of the ventilator and put him in our hands, his body started turning blue. All of our family members started uttering the mantras for the last rites. But suddenly, my son's body started turning pink! This allowed the doctors to begin treatment again and the next day, the doctors said that my baby survived.

The hospital neurologist and medical team said that though he survived, he would struggle his entire life. He would make our family struggle. We would have marital fights surrounding his life. Worry, anxiety, and anger would stem from his existence. Constantly they were saying that he would not be able to walk, talk, or eat like a normal kid. They diagnosed him with cerebral palsy (damage to the developing brain that affects a person's ability to control their muscles) and epilepsy (a brain disorder characterized by repeated seizures). They predicted he would be a vegetable, his life expectancy would not be beyond 40, and that he would have life-long complications.

Three years prior, in 1995, after becoming an assistant vice president at a German bank, I endured a life-threatening experience of Steven-Johnson Syndrome, marked by severe viral symptoms and skin rashes, which led to a critical hospital transfer and a challenging recovery. This made me realize the value of life, so I said it was okay even if my son would be a vegetable for his entire life. I just wanted my son to be alive, and I would take care of my son. This fire began to spread in my heart, and I thought, if I cry any more, I'll be taken over by depression and lose my ability to function effectively. There will be no one to take care of my son. So I got myself ready for this challenge.

From that day forward, day after day, love was in the air surrounding my son. Through the challenges, he thrived, he was a fighter and a warrior because love is a choice. I chose to love this child and raise him the best that I know how, but it doesn't negate the pain that also marinates within when faced with the truth of the situation. I realized that being the mom of a child with special needs requires a unique strength. And the way I viewed the world changed. I started seeing on this journey that the community and the world around him had lower expectations for my child, and I realized how little effort people will put into communicating with a child in his situation.

Even though we had become U.S. citizens, my strong Indian accent persisted, and I could feel prejudice and disparities shown in therapy treatments and in services throughout my son's various life phases. I had to struggle to advocate for my son's rights in the public school system and inclusion in the general education classroom in addition to finding a community center that would accept a child with multiple special needs. Nevertheless, I persisted. I decided to build my own network of support with a lot of friends and lots of activities. I built an extended family of people who understood the aches of my child and wanted to genuinely connect with him. Defeat was not an option, and when hope abounds, love will triumph.

I also started to see that approaching experts was always expensive and the only way we could financially access them was through insurance in the United States. I decided to gain knowledge in therapy treatments and modalities to help my son with support at home and also started to help other kids with disabilities and their parents.

And although I struggled due to my ethnic background and accent, I completed my master's degree in special education and behavioral analysis and became a certified autism specialist just to help my son and other children and families. Persistence and success can conquer challenges.

My son is now a 25-year-old happy man who has cerebral palsy and is currently living in his own home with support. Although he experiences challenges, some of the most fulfilling moments are watching him exceed other people's expectations, meet milestones we thought he would never meet, and flourish in his small-scale business, called Athish Handi Kreations. With the help of his attendants, he is shattering the world's limits and thriving. He proved that his diagnosis does not define him.

My inspiration in life since my childhood was Mother Teresa. I always wanted to follow Mother Teresa's humility, simplicity, and helping nature with the underprivileged. She had such a simple approach to the most complex problems in life. I have learned from her life that it is much easier to accomplish something when you have one agenda. We all have one life to live, and I want to do as much as I can with my time. So, I decided to focus on making a difference in the lives of the families of children and adults with disabilities.

In my early parenting days, joining parents of special needs support groups with a focus on cerebral palsy and South Asian origin helped refine my parenting skills and reset my expectations for my child, enhancing my sense of competence. Engaging with other parents broadened my perspective, helping me envision a hopeful future for my son, with new ideas gradually reshaping my outlook. I've also seen Indian-origin parents yearning for such interactions due to cultural and linguistic hurdles. Regular meetings, whether in person or through social media, uncovered challenges tied to cultural diversity, family dynamics, and personal constraints like time, transportation, and childcare.

Desiring to connect and share knowledge with other Indian families of children with special needs, I began forming support groups for Indian parents and parents of special needs on Facebook and WhatsApp. This led parents, including me, towards a sense of belonging, feeling more confident and empowered in addressing our children's disabilities. We were able to share common challenges immigrant families face related to cultural prejudice, accessing services, balancing work, life, and caregiving, and dealing with social and internal family pressures related to raising a child with special needs. The moral support within these groups significantly alleviates feelings of isolation, loneliness, and guilt, making interactions more equitable and less discriminatory. This parent-to-parent support has morphed into a familial bond among members, where emotional support and valuable information flow freely, enriching our experience as parents of children with special needs.

Hosting these groups emerged as a high priority for my husband and me, and I established WeEMBRACE, in 2018 as a registered 501(c)(3) nonprofit organization. The focus is to support individuals of varying abilities and their families, advocating for inclusion and equal opportunities. Initially, a support mechanism for South Asian families of

Indian, Chinese, Korean, Filipino, and American origin, it has evolved significantly and now offers numerous virtual and physical classes, adaptive sports, a unique buddy match program, and annual events like talent shows and sports days which raise community awareness. The vision is expanding, with plans for a dedicated center offering a range of classes, a sensory lab, vocational training for adults, and wellness activities. This center also aims to be a respite for parents, providing empowerment through educational meetings. Through WeEMBRACE, we've created a vital, growing community platform.

As a result of my experiences, I am a lot more patient and have more of an open mind when facing challenges. I want to change the world for the better. I have learned to be a strong advocate for my child and for other children who are neurodivergent. No one knows my child better than I do, and I have learned to trust that. Giving to others helped to protect my mental and physical health, has reduced my stress levels, kept me mentally stimulated, and provided a sense of purpose.

This special journey at different stages of my life has helped me grow spiritually. I believe in The Bhagavad Gita which has helped me get answers to three fundamental questions:

1. Who am I?
2. What am I doing here?
3. What should I do next?

I remind myself of the teachings of The Gita to bring harmony within myself, harmony in dealing with others, and harmony with the world I live in.

I used to follow The Bhagavad Gita teachings in my previous life, even before my child was born. This has helped me to be detached from outcomes and simply focus on doing my duty. While I am fighting with my daily challenges, I learned to treat victory and defeat, pleasure, and pain as the same.

My Recommendations

Drawing from my journey to becoming a parent of an adult child, as well as my continuous learning and guidance from mentors and life experiences, I humbly offer these personal insights to you:

1. Try something new. It sounds simple but you may find yourself in a rut with a therapy schedule that is not producing results, or a therapist/provider that is not a good fit. Do not be afraid to try new people or approaches until you find the right fit for your child.

2. Be prepared to accept that the best fit may change, and you will need to try something new again. It may be that your child "failed" at something other kids can do but pay close attention to how and why they had trouble. This information is essential to helping your child move forward and it gives the provider team insight about where to focus future treatment plans.

3. Find a community of parents who are facing similar challenges that you can relate to and have

conversations with them regularly. You will need this support in your entire journey, and you can also share the same with someone else and make their life better.

4. Embrace the diagnosis when you're ready, but remember your child is *your* child. Don't look at your baby the way the world does. Don't set limitations on them because of the label they are given. Believe in your child, believe in yourself as their parent, and remember to always be their advocate and voice. Our children can and will do incredible things if we don't let negativity and doubt intrude on their lives. Teach your child they can do and be anything and that the label doesn't define who they are. Remember to have and give grace, to your child and to yourself. Remember your child doesn't need to change, but do everything in your power to change the world FOR THEM.

My Wish for You

"All kids need is a little help, a little hope, and someone who believes in them."

- Magic Johnson.

All children need belief, hope, and support, especially those with special needs. As parents of these unique kids, our challenges differ, but our core desires remain the same: love, acceptance, and understanding, both for us and our children. Raising a child with special needs isn't merely about addressing their challenges but about cherishing their strengths. It demands resilience and tenacity. We, parents, are driven to create a joyful world for them, fueled by unwavering hope. Our children's happiness becomes our guiding force. I urge everyone to increase awareness, understand, and empathize with families like ours. To all who read this, remember: love unconditionally, refrain from judgment, and always be kind. To fellow parents on this journey: you aren't alone. Let's stand together in support.

Ways to Connect with Me

These are the ways to connect with me and WeEMBRACE.

Website: www.weembracefamilies.org

LinkedIn: www.linkedin.com/in/nkmeena

Facebook: https://www.facebook.com/Meenakalyanasundaram/

You tube: https://www.youtube.com/@WeEMBRACE

WhatsApp: https://chat.whatsapp.com/EHFcrWdicCR5I7tyWS7hfU

Meena Kalyanasundaram is a mother of a 25-year-old young man with cerebral palsy and epilepsy. Meena Kalyanasundaram is a strong advocate for her son and other children and adults like her son. She and her husband, Somasundaram, founded WeEMBRACE in 2018 and a microenterprise, Athish Handi Kreations. They have struggled to get the services and support needed to improve their son's quality of life despite his challenges and hardships. WeEMBRACE is a nonprofit organization, which serves more than 200 families of neuro-diverse individuals in and around Sacramento, CA, and more than 500 families nationwide.

Cerebral Palsy Foundation - https://www.yourcpf.org/

Epilepsy - Epilepsy Foundation - https://www.epilepsy.com/what-is-epilepsy

When Being Different Makes a Difference

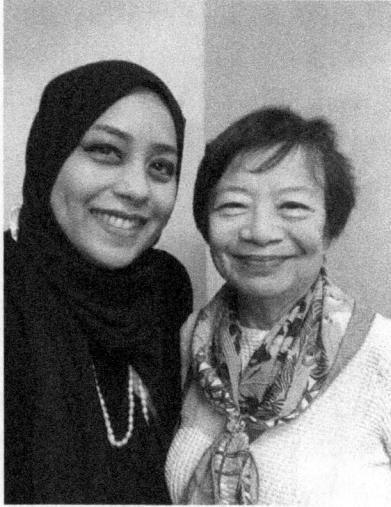

Nadhiya Ito, M.A., CCC-SLP

伊藤ナディヤ

This year (2023) marks my 18th year of being a speech-language pathologist (SLP). My passion for my work remains unchanged after all these years. This has been a journey of learning, not only the academics and how to be a good therapist, but also about empathy, compassion, connection, empowerment, advocacy, and personal growth, both as an individual and as a clinician. Making a

Becoming an Exceptional API Leader

difference has always been my motivation, and it was definitely one of the reasons why I chose to become an SLP. Throughout this journey, I have also come to realize that I am who I am today because of the people who made a difference in my life.

Having a Sri Lankan father and a Japanese mother, I was born and raised in Japan until I was almost 14. Of course, my younger brother and I looked different from the rest of our Japanese friends, but growing up in Tokyo, we were fortunate to have been surrounded by other children, who were also "half" (ハーフ), i.e., half-Japanese or "mixed," like us. As a child, I always internally identified myself as a Japanese individual, because that was all I knew myself to be. It was not until later that I realized that others perceived us differently because of how we looked. I remember being picked on by some kids in elementary school for being a "foreigner" or *gaijin* (外人). As a child, this was very confusing to me. I knew my father was a gaijin, but me? Japan was all I knew, and I only spoke Japanese. Luckily, I had many wonderful friends who always defended me. My amazing teachers also often reminded me that, "We live in an international world, and you should be proud of who you are."

When you grow up in a homogeneous and collective society like Japan, you try to fit in and not stand out, especially as a young child. Growing up as a mixed child in Japan, I do not believe I valued my difference as something that was positive. In fact, there is even a proverb in Japan, "出る杭は打たれる" (*Deru kui wa*

104

utareru), literally meaning, "The stake that stands out gets hammered down." Basically: "If you stand out, you will be subject to criticism," or "Difference is forced into conformity." I remember subconsciously thinking as I was growing up that I didn't want to be different from the rest of my friends. Yet, I was very different, not only in the way I looked, but I also did things to stand out, such as being on a student council or playing a main role in a play!

When I was 13, my family experienced the sudden demise of our father. Subsequently, my Japanese mother decided to move us to Sri Lanka (a country we had previously visited only 3 times!), so my brother and I could learn about our father's country, religion, languages, and cultures and, most importantly, so we could spend time with our paternal side of the family. As you can imagine, this was a significant transition for all of us. We did not speak English, Sinhala, or Tamil, the three languages spoken in Sri Lanka, so there was an issue with communication. Not being able to communicate your thoughts in a manner you are used to doing in your native language was definitely a challenge for us. Although our father was a polyglot who knew eight languages (i.e., English, Tamil, Sinhala, Japanese, Hindi, French, German, and Korean), he only spoke to us in Japanese. In Sri Lanka, my brother and I attended an international school, and as a result, English became our second language. I subsequently learned/studied Tamil, Sinhala, and French, and also learned to read Arabic to read the Quran. I remember carrying five different dictionaries to school every day (and this was before the days of having access to Google translate!). My love for languages, I believe, is something I innately inherited from my father. While I consider only Japanese and English to be my clinical languages—the languages I feel competent to use in my SLP practice—I continue to work on improving the others, in addition to sign language (Signed Exact English and ASL) and Spanish, which I learned after moving to the United States. Hopefully, someday, I will become proficient enough to use many of them in my clinical practice. I know that this will open doors to connecting with more clients and families that come from diverse backgrounds. Being multilingual, as you can imagine, is a highly sought skill as an SLP, especially when working in a diverse city like ours, Los Angeles.

In Sri Lanka, I was called the "Japanese girl" (and I knew everyone meant well by calling me so). To them, I did not look Sri Lankan enough. Even when I decided to wear a hijab, a head covering or a scarf for Muslim women, at age 16, I was the "Japanese girl with a hijab." Have you ever met a Japanese Hijabi (besides me) before? Chances are that you haven't, and perhaps, you won't forget about me! An interesting thing is that we live in a world where our looks no longer match the languages we speak or the cultures we identify with. It always amuses me to be spoken to in English at a Japanese bookstore, when I'm, in fact, buying books written in Japanese. My appearance, especially my hijab, precedes the notion that perhaps I am a native and fluent Japanese speaker!

My journey of exploring my own identity has been an interesting one, especially as a mixed person. I am Japanese. I am Sri Lankan. I am now an American. I am also a Muslim (which is evident because of my Hijab). And

Nadhiya Ito

I am Asian. Based on my diversified life experiences and identity, being able to relate to others who come from diverse linguistic and cultural backgrounds has truly been a gift, although I did not realize it until much later in life.

My journey as a prospective SLP began when I met a Caucasian lady on a public bus in Sri Lanka, when I was a senior in high school. I had never traveled on a bus alone in Sri Lanka prior to this, and sitting next to this foreigner in an empty bus was such an unusual experience for me. (At that time, you did not typically see a foreigner on a bus, unless you were my mother(!)). The lady and I happened to have a conversation, and she told me that she was a speech therapist from the UK and that she was there to help set up the country's first and only speech therapy program. What is speech therapy? I had no idea. She shared with me how fulfilling her work was and that there was only one speech therapist in the entire country at that time.

I went home to research online and the rest is history. Meeting this lady, who, many years later, I found out to be Dr. Mary Wickenden, was a pivotal moment in my life because it led me to pursue my career as an SLP. You may find it interesting to know that I found her contact information online almost 23 years later and wrote to her to tell her that she was the reason I became an SLP. To my surprise, she immediately wrote back to me and confirmed that she lived in Sri Lanka at that time and that she traveled by bus to get to places. While she did not recall meeting me on the bus, she did say that it was quite likely that it was her, given the circumstances. It made me cry to read her words saying that *if* it was indeed her, she was very glad that she influenced my career choice and that it all worked out well. Our encounter was very brief yet so impactful. Dr. Wickenden made a huge difference in my life.

Upon graduating from high school, I moved to the United States to attend Missouri State University, where I completed my bachelor of science degree in communication sciences and disorders (speech-language pathology). At that time, I was one of over 500 international students and one of the only four Hijabis on campus. Of course, I stood out. It made it rather difficult, especially when 9/11 happened and there was an increased sense of patriotism on campus, which prompted all the international students to feel isolated and not welcome. It heightened my sense of what it was like to be a minority. I was elected to be the president of the Association of International Students and, subsequently, was invited as the only student speaker to share my experience and perspectives at the 9/11 memorial service on campus the following year. I was very nervous, but when I look back, what an amazing opportunity it was to represent my fellow international students and the Muslim community! Yes, representation matters! This was just the beginning.

In 2002, my senior year in college, I attended my first American Speech-Language Hearing Association (ASHA) convention in Atlanta, GA. This was when I saw an Asian lady (Taiwanese, to be precise) walking by, and I immediately recognized her as Dr. Lilly Cheng, as I had read her article in one of our classes before. In my mind, she represented the Asians in our field, and that meant a lot to me. Star-struck, I ran after her. I introduced myself, and she took time to talk to me. She invited me to my first Asian Pacific Islander Speech-Language-Hearing Caucus (thereafter, the API Caucus) meeting, which she chaired, and I was blown away by her passionate words. She said, "Because of your background, there will be people who can benefit from your services."

It really resonated with me, and I slowly began to see the notion of being a "minority" as my strength. Her words were truly empowering. I applied to pursue my master's degree in communicative disorders at San Diego State University, and Dr. Cheng became my professor and, later, my mentor. She continues to make a difference in my life, including providing me with an opportunity to share my story by writing this chapter in this book.

I became involved in the API Caucus as a student, and later served as a caucus Secretary and the vice president. Twenty-one years after I attended my first API caucus meeting, I currently serve as an advisory board member. I am truly proud of the work we, as an organization, have accomplished thus far and continue to do. Being able to connect, share experiences and stories, collaborate, and be of service to the clients, families, students, and professionals of API background has truly been a rewarding experience.

Representation truly matters. Throughout my career as an SLP, I have worked at Los Angeles Speech & Language Therapy Center, a diverse private practice, founded by Dr. Pamela Wiley in 1979, when she saw a disparity in the services our minority children were receiving. At the clinic, I have had an opportunity to work with clients and families who look like me—someone who is of mixed race, who dresses like me, who communicates with the same languages, or who share similar cultural backgrounds. Being or feeling represented provides a sense of belonging. When the clients and the families can see themselves in us, externally or internally, it creates an extra layer of connectedness that aids in the therapeutic process.

It is, however, important to note that across the United States, API populations are significantly underrepresented among speech, language, and hearing professionals and make up only 2.8% of the entire membership of ASHA, according to the ASHA Member & Affiliate Profile (2022). The dire need for professionals in our field who represent our clients and their families cannot be stressed enough. We have unique needs, and an understanding of our cultures and languages is warranted for effective outcomes.

Had it not been for the realization that "being different" can be a positive attribute in touching other people's lives, I may still have considered myself inferior in my chosen career field due to my differences. Being different can mean a variety of things. Not only does it include differences in culture and languages, but also family dynamics, socioeconomics, religious beliefs, neurodiversity, gender, skill sets, life experiences, perspectives, and even a disability. You may "stand out" because of these differences, especially if you are part of a homogeneous and collective community, and this may sometimes prompt someone to be regarded unfairly. Working with the API population, I have come across families who were going through such cultural dilemmas when it came to disability, ranging from not being able to introduce their child to his/her grandparents due to an autism diagnosis, or families declining psychological consultations due to fears that the potential diagnosis (i.e., being different from the peers) would lead to discrimination within the community and eventually hinder him/her from being employed as an adult. While we may not be able to make a drastic change in the lives of our clients and their families, I know that given my background, I have the potential to be their advocate and assist them in navigating through their journey.

Life in America can be complex, especially when you live back and forth between collective and individualistic societies. Facing the unknown can be a scary experience, regardless of what your cultural background may be. A Japanese parent once said this to me. "My daughter is Japanese, but she is also American, and she will continue to live here. I want her to grow up valuing her Japanese culture and heritage, but I also want her to be able to navigate life in America as well and be as independent as possible." As an SLP, I often wonder what I can do and how I can contribute so that when we target communication, our clients can soar in both worlds successfully.

Being different can make a difference, and although this is still rather a new notion, it is an important one for me.

Once an intern said to me, "I think I made a difference today." I looked at him and couldn't help but smile. I cannot explain enough how much those words resonated with me. The truth is that the process of making a difference is a subconscious act of service. You may have the intention of making a difference but the act itself comes from your heart. You follow your passion; you follow what you believe in, and everything happens in the moment. If you are lucky, you may realize later that you've touched the lives of other people. It's not only a good feeling, but it also keeps you going. It makes you a better clinician and a better person.

I still have a lot to learn, but the opportunities presented to me, thus far, to serve my clients and my community as an advocate in communication, while embracing my differences as my strength, have affirmed that I'm doing what I was destined to do.

My Recommendations

Here are some of my personal recommendations as you consider being involved and contributing to the API community:

- Be involved—If you are of API background, share cultures, and/or speak one or more API languages, we need you! As Dr. Lilly Cheng said, "Because of your background, there will be people who can benefit from your services."

- Be our ally!—You don't have to be of API descent to contribute. You can always be our ally! If you have an interest, knowledge, or understanding of API languages or cultures, know that people will appreciate everything you can offer. We need people like you, who are compassionate and want to make a difference.

- Ask questions—Get to know our cultures, languages, and our ways of life, and don't hesitate to ask questions if you are not sure. Although the API population is often regarded as one group, there is so much diversity among our communities. Get to know us! Let's learn together!

My Wish for You

Whether you are a therapist, an educator, a caregiver, a family member, or even a friend, whatever your role in your life may be, I hope you know that you bring value based on your differences. If it's not you, then, who?

I hope you continue to make a difference.

"With gratitude to all those who made a difference in my life."

– Nadhiya

Ways to Connect with Me

https://linktr.ee/Nadhiya_Treasured.Adornment

Email: nadhiya@yahoo.com

Instagram: @treasuredadornment

LinkedIn: https://www.linkedin.com/in/nadhiyaito/

Nadhiya Ito, M.A., CCC-SLP is a speech-language pathologist and a clinical supervisor at Los Angeles Speech & Language Therapy Center, in California. She is a past vice president and a current advisory board member of the Asian Pacific Islander Speech-Language Hearing Caucus, where she has been an active member for the past 21 years. She is a native speaker of Japanese and provides bilingual (Japanese-English) services. Working at a family-centered private practice for the past 18 years, Nadhiya is passionate about empowering and advocating for clients and families, especially the culturally and linguistically diverse populations.

Multilingual Multitudes

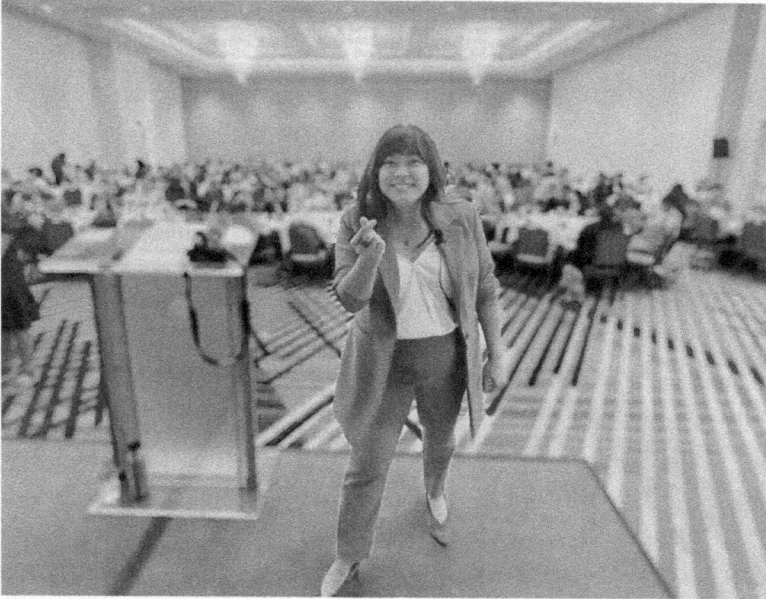

Phương Liên Palafox, CCC-SLP

連及方

Bilingual Betrayal

Kids hold secrets—lying about brushing their teeth or taking an extra *bánh ngọt*. As an immigrant kid, the hush-hush hides an entire home existence. So, I buried my Vietnamese upon entry into kindergarten. Hiding, though, is a thing of exhaustion. Over time, these efforts swelled into shame for my family's language of expression. For self-preservation, I trusted the world and glorified English—each syllable executed with fervor, biting my teeth tightly to hold the /s/ sound that conveys plurality and memorizing so-many versions of English verbs. Alas, with all buried truths, the cost is cancerous. Despite the grand effort to cloak my otherness, my days (and face) were visibly Asian. And, it was eating me from the outside-in.

Age 6: My kindergarten teacher told *Má* I needed to transfer to the school across town. I did not speak that year, and it was assumed I did not understand the version of English spoken in class. I understood everything.

Age 8: "Color the action words that were taught to you," my first-grade teacher said, while handing out a worksheet. I stared at the paper confused. I walked up to her desk and asked, "What 'taught' means?" Verbs are not conjugated in Vietnamese. She stood up and called the class to attention, "Class, can anyone tell Phuong what 'taught' means?" I felt stupid, and my teacher made sure my entire class knew it.

Age 15: As I walked down the hall between classes, I saw an upperclassman. We were friends. He smiled, started parting the masses of students with his arms and projected, "PHUONG! Make waaaaaay. Chink-chong-Phuong coming through!" He laughed, gave me an affirming nod, and continued to project human confetti throughout the hallway as he walked to class. I reciprocated his laugh feeling simultaneously acknowledged and rejected.

There's more. I've lived 15,752 days, and 41.5% of this time has included my roles and responsibilities as an educator and service provider. Of late, I have begun to reflect upon the memories made within the last two decades in my field of speech and language sciences. It is within this quiet, nuanced space that I have begun to see the dark thread tethering my professional days.

For too many hours, I gave my work my trust. In return, I was bestowed a contract that required relinquishment of my family's language, necessary conformity, and existence as an (English-) grammar fanatic.

The murk I felt as I sat in small mirrored rooms observed by supervisors, walked through university hallways, waited in IEP rooms, assessed in classroom spaces, and stood in presentation halls left its slimy trail on my narrative as a bilingual, bicultural Vietnamese-Chinese American. I understood, finally, my unwillingness to move past the shiny exterior of my work. Self-preservation, at times, is the sole medicine to fuel the seasons of our lives. With time and privilege, I deliberately exposed the grime. Oh, the memories I found—some polished for the sake of levity, some wrapped in layers of naïveté, some hard-pressed and repressed.

Age 23: A clinical supervisor held my report covered in red edits and said I wrote poorly because English was not my first language.

Age 35: An educator pulled me aside following a meeting to say, "I just don't know how you do it. Your English is SO GOOD!"

Age 36: A colleague told me, following a state presentation to thousands, that I mispronounced a word.

Every age: There have been too many microaggressions about my name, Phuong. "I am not even going to try to say that." "What's your American name?" On the day I went to vote during my lunch break, as the voting volunteer took my driver's license to confirm my address, she stated, "Oh, that's an interesting name." I ignored her comment. "Really. Such an interesting name." I stated, "It's actually a common name where my family grew up." She quickly retorted, "Well, where *I* come from, it's *interesting*." As I stood in line to carry out my civic duties, my eyes got wet.

I thought about how *Ba*, a South Vietnamese naval captain and prisoner of war, navigated a wooden boat with my *má* and 54 other refugees across the South China Sea. I thought about how it was safer for my parents to step onto water than to stay on Vietnamese land. I thought about how they landed in Hong Kong's harbor after several weeks of hunger. I thought about how I was born at 3 a.m. that very morning. I thought about how *Má* had given me the name Phương. I thought about how she often told me it means "going in the right direction."

There is nothing small about microaggressions. Each cut hurts, and I feel like I'm moving through this earth, some days, completely raw.

Multilingual Exaltation

Now, I spend my 45-year-old days as a bilingual speech-language therapist in the United States. My work honors sounds and language structures of faraway places. I walk alongside families, school districts, and organizations to empower dual language learners. This

118

shift, from living my own bicultural life to moving alongside others' lives, was much-needed "oxygen" to awaken worthy, bilingual me. What has been uncovered within me in the last two decades is unapologetic fire and fervor for multilingual communicators.

In this professional space, I observed the same sentiments—English ruled. It was used to develop tests to determine others' communication abilities. It was on all intake forms. It was the sole language of testing when deciding if a student needed an Individualized Education Plan for special education—regardless of the student's language(s) of exposure. Families were (wrongly) told to communicate in English to support academic and communication success by educational and medical professionals… despite what the research stated.

Multilingual needs are not just for students, clients, and patients. This also applies to the bilingual, bicultural educators and service providers, too. My 20+ years have unveiled that societal and professional spaces require, utilize, and, ultimately, exploit multilingual communicators. I have observed caseloads for bilingual speech-language specialists that are significantly higher than their English-only speaking professional peers. Additionally, because the work requires execution in two or more languages, the tasks take twice as long with fewer resources. I also witness bilingual professionals being asked to support bilingual efforts (e.g., interpreting, translating, diversity-equity-inclusion-efforts) that are not a part of their hired responsibilities. The outcomes of such profiteering are a cruel complement to the aforementioned censorship of multilingualism.

These are personal aggressions that I've digested for too long, and it has been making me sick. Being told that I cannot serve the bilingual Vietnamese campus in my district as one of the few Vietnamese-American speech-language specialists in my state feels discounting for my Vietnamese community. Being told that I need to help with additional duties for my bilingualism without compensation, though meaningful, feels exhausting. Being questioned about the "proficiency" of my heritage language when the responsibility of supporting multilingual communities, by law, is the responsibility of all educators and medical professionals, feels discriminatory. Being asked to share my stories in presentations and written publications without compensation feels icky. And, please let it be known, that all of these aches exist alongside the multilingual good, the multilingual gifts, and the multilingual joy. Being able to spend my earthly days advocating for multilingual rights is a privilege I get to execute.

My Sacred Gifts

As I looked back on my narrative, truths were unveiled. My environment, swathed in centering the majority language, led me astray. The autonomy of adulthood has regifted me with my sacred Việt sounds, words, and stories. These medicinal lived experiences, coincidentally, are the fastening between my past and sacred agency to fuel the future of our multilingual communities. Oh, there is so much gratitude I have for the following personal, spiritual, and community gifts:

- **Engage in Educational Opportunities** to invest in learning experiences alongside others have contributed in meaningful ways. First, I get to empower families to communicate, in words or gestures or visuals, their heritage language. Through my lens, this singular act has given families the permission they needed to revel in their language and culture to immerse in their authentic bicultural narrative. Second, I get to spend time with professional peers to invest in human-centered ways to support heritage languages and communication access.

- **Recognize the Representation** by sharing all the parts of me, my simple existence has been disrupting systems within the field of communication sciences. Showing up has provided representation for Asian Pacific Islander students and professionals. I do not take for granted invitations to be the first Asian-American to exist in spaces—school district leadership, regional leadership, and keynotes for state conferences. Through mentorship representation, I get to be what I did not have. While many may assume this is a hierarchical relationship, experience has shown me the gifts of such a relationship feed both parties, and I am grateful. Finally, I created a scholarship at my alma mater, The University of Texas at Austin. The annual funds would be provided to a bilingual graduate student. In 2023, the first recipient of the Phương Liên Palafox Scholarship was awarded. This act is an example of how representation ultimately yields necessary representation.

- **Collective Camaraderie.** An unexpected gift of providing professional development has been the community I have found alongside my bilingual, bicultural peers. The truth is that being bilingual is a complicated thing. For many of us, it's not just about the language. It's also about living. Being bilingual is communicating in two languages. Being bicultural is existing within two cultures, two worlds. The difference is making a choice to study a language versus needing to cram one for survival. I know that my healing has been the direct result of the understanding, empathy, and big-love from individuals who have digested similar stories.

- **Generational Joy.** This past spring, my siblings, their children, my *Ba*, and I sat in a crowded cafeteria at Summitt Elementary School in the Austin Independent School District. We were there to watch my 7-year-old perform in their annual *Tết*, Lunar New Year, show at the only Vietnamese two-way dual-language program in the world. Above my father's head hung the flag of South Vietnam. As the drums began and the lions emerged down the aisles, tears came to my eyes again. The wet path down my Asian face, this time, hydrated decades of cultural drought. We don't recognize the light without existing in the dark, and it was so very bright that evening. From this purview, I look back at little-Phương with so much love. I understand that she existed within generational trauma, and the aftermath of this is also generational resilience.

- **Peace in the Process.** Finally, as I do this work alongside my communities, there are moments that hold very big feelings. There are outcomes that anger and carry so much sadness. I am grateful to carry this work, *and* it is very heavy. As a highly sensitive person with daily crying, I have learned about finding peace in this whole process of working and living. I fuel myself first. I exercise my body, protect my bandwidth, meditate, and rest. Then, I give from my overflow.

My Recommendations: Multilingual Magic

My intention is to color our world with the following sentiments:

- English-only ideologies have historically prevailed in parts of the world, and this has squelched heritage languages. Multilingualism is not a pathology despite the crescendo of commentary during my lifetime. There are more than 100 languages within Asian Pacific Islander communities, and every single member has a right to access equitable educational opportunities and medical care.

- Give students, clients, patients, and families permission to communicate in their heritage languages. Share this message explicitly. I can report with research that giving families permission to communicate in their heritage language supports academic success and boosts communication progress. Most importantly, it honors the family's worthy cultural narrative.

- Get names right. A name is the most important character in a story that individual is living. Say, "Your name is important. I want to get it right." Then, practice and use the name. Finally, mistakes happen. Apologize and try again. The honor is not in the avoidance of an error. The honor is in the trying and trying and trying again because the person is worth the effort.

- There is no such thing as "good English." When people apologize for their communication, I respond with, "Your English is perfect. It represents a faraway place that is important." As multilingual communicators, we are products of our experiences, and binary thoughts of "good" or "bad" expressive language use are fabricated. There is no "correct" value of knowing a language. People have judged my Vietnamese. I attended school in the United States and did not have Vietnamese within my educational programming. We all have our language exposures, and it is all worthy. I'm the product of a meaningful narrative, and I am the amazing outcome. Such ideas hold multilingual communicators to unfair expectations and standards when, ego aside, we already know more than the monolingual communicator.

My Gift to You

As I think about my intentions for this chapter contribution, I go back to centering the power of stories. For readers who want to invest in allyship and agency for supporting Asian Pacific Islander communities, I wish for you the gift of digesting lived experiences of API narratives. Exist alongside these tales and revel in the feelings that are shared. Within this space, I want you to know that you can make meaningful connections. Many individuals have honored my days as an Asian-American Pacific Islander, and every single one of these moments is secured together by intentional action to care about my authentic well-being.

And, finally, to my bilingual, bicultural humans, I want you to know that I understand. I see you existing within two (or more) worlds, and you are perfect just as you are. You hold many settings within your days, and I know the weight of this can be substantive. Your value, your worth is not based on how much you know and use your family's language. These are fabricated criteria that do not consider historical events that contribute to families moving across the world. You are a part of and a product of our history.

Thank you for supporting your parents and caregivers when they were navigating new settings.

Thank you for being mentors for newer generations despite not having them in your own life.

Thank you for sharing all the parts of you alongside the prevalence of our majority language.

Thank you for showing up, day after day, and sharing your representation and light.

To those of us who are multilingual, we are exponentially perfect holding and honoring all parts of us. Here's to being worthy.

Ways to Connect with Me

I look forward to connecting with you.

www.phuonglienpalafox.com

Email: connect@phuonglienpalafox.com

Instagram: @PhuongLienPalafox

Facebook: PhuongLienPalafoxSLP

Phương Liên Palafox (she/her) is a Vietnamese-Chinese multilingual speech-language scientist, author and advocate. She has worked within and alongside school districts for the last two decades. Currently, her time is spent empowering clients and their families in her clinic, and she provides training and keynotes for educational and state organizations. With a foundation of evidence-based, human-centered practices, she invests in culturally responsive and sustaining practices, narrative-based interventions and advocacy for educators and service providers. She is the author of *The Heartbeat of Speech-Language Pathology*. Attendees leave her presentations and storytelling feeling validated, refueled, and re-engaged in their already-impactful, meaningful work.

Walking into a Wonderful Life

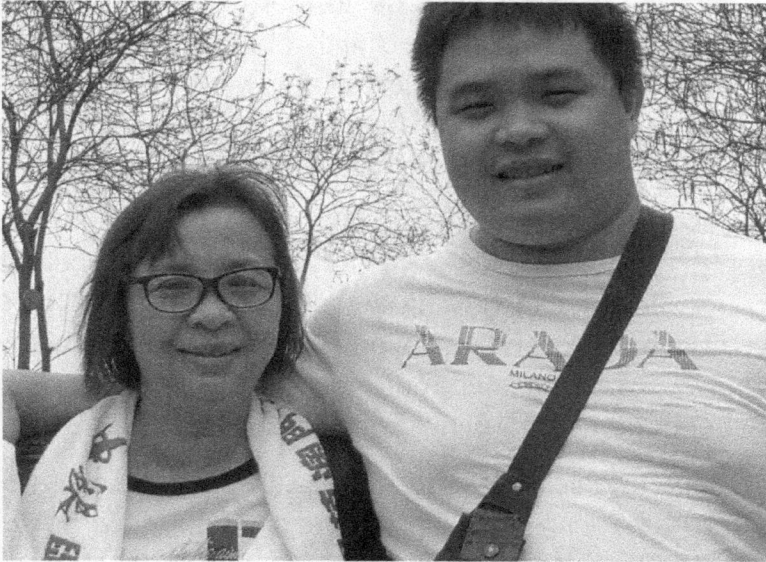

Lou Sio Ha, Ruby

盧紹霞

A single mother in Macau, I am currently 68 years old, and my son is 39. The past three decades have been a long journey of patience, empowerment, and teamwork. I share my experiences as the mother of an autistic child in hopes of helping other families in similar situations.

I was told by the doctor that Antonio had an "autistic tendency" when he was nine months old. When I heard the term, I was not sure what it meant. But I knew it would be challenging, something my husband and I would have to face. As a toddler, Antonio exhibited several symptoms: it took him longer than average to learn how to speak, he was not interested in playing with other children, and he had emotional outbursts, such as throwing tissues out the window. Antonio was later diagnosed with severe autism when he was three years old in 1987.

Autism is a developmental disorder with three levels of severity. Those with severe autism require substantial support and tend to be characterized by a lack of verbal and nonverbal communication skills, difficulty handling changing routines, extreme focus, a limited desire for social engagement, and disruptive behavior.

When Antonio was diagnosed with severe autism, we had to enroll him in a special school for children with autism in Hong Kong, because there was no such school in Macau at that time. Fortunately, my husband's sister is a Hong Kong resident, and she offered to take care of him in Hong Kong so I could keep my job in Macau.

I was worried about how he would be accepted and was deeply concerned about how he would interact at school. I also felt uneasy about leaving him in the care of my sister-in-law and felt guilty about not being with him every day to care for him as his mother. I visited Antonio most weekends until we moved him back to Macau in 1991 when the Concordia School for Special Education in Macau started to offer education to children with intellectual disabilities. He was about seven years old at that time. My sister-in-law and her family helped me take care of him and always welcomed him at family gatherings so he could learn how to interact with people. This was extremely helpful to his development. Their support continued after my husband and I got divorced in 1995 when Antonio turned 11. For that, I am very grateful.

Shortly after the divorce, I drove myself very hard at work to distract myself from the sadness of being a single mother and a divorcee. Then one day, I received a call from Antonio's teacher, asking me if something bad had happened to our family because he started lying on the ground at school. This was the way Antonio expressed his unhappiness. Children with autism often express their emotions and insecurity through various disruptive behaviors. That day, I realized that my emotions were having a strong influence on my son, but he did not express his feelings to me because he did not want to worry me.

I started doing a lot of volunteer work to fill myself with positive energy, and in 1998 I became a board member of Talent of People Charity Association of Macau. From 2002 to 2018, Antonio and I joined the volunteer team of Talent to visit underprivileged students living in the mountainous regions of China. These meaningful experiences had a great impact on us. We realized that compared to a lot of people, we were very blessed and should cherish everything we have. To reward society, Antonio and I began to sponsor some underprivileged students to complete their high school education in 2007. We are so happy that they are all now working in society and have their own families. We still keep in contact with some of them.

Children with autism often have emotional issues. For instance, when Antonio was younger, he would bite his fingers and jump around if he heard a sudden, loud noise. It was not too bad when he was just a child. But as he grew older and bigger, this behavior at times scared people. As parents of children with autism, we need to help our children understand that this is not their fault; however, their emotions can affect other people. As a Chinese woman, I was taught to be respectful of others, and I was concerned that his behaviors would bother other people. So we need to keep reminding our children to control their emotions and help them make progress step by step.

In 2018, a social worker we consulted told Antonio that the voices [his unstable emotions] are actually "the little elf" living in his body. The counselor encouraged him to learn to get along with the little elf and not to be influenced by it. This inspired him to create his illustrated book called *The Elf in My Body*, published in 2019 with the support of Shenmo Education, depicting how autistic people calm their emotions.

It is always difficult to find ways to communicate emotions at the beginning. As long as we find a way to communicate with our children, things get much easier with time.

I believe that if we give our children trust and opportunities, they will go very far in life, and I also believe that every person has many ways to succeed—we do not need to just focus on a career or making money. As

Antonio grew older, I encouraged him to try out different hobbies, from swimming to music and painting. After finishing secondary school at the Concordia School for Special Education in Macau in 2006, Antonio joined the Special Olympics World Summer Games, and in 2007, he won a number of medals for freestyle swimming. In 2011, he also became the captain and marimba player of the Sunny Band (the first musical band formed by autistic and intellectually disabled people in Macau). In December 2019, Shenmo Education invited Antonio to host a launch event in Beijing for his book, where he had a chance to share his experience of living with autism.

Before I retired in 2012, I set up some investment plans, so we could continue to receive a stable income. Now, I am able to spend a lot of time with Antonio every day, teaching him every little detail about our daily life and helping him be independent. Since then, I started giving him more responsibilities, starting with preparing breakfast for the two of us every day. Not only does he need to cook meals, but he also has to buy the ingredients. In this way, he was able to learn about the concept of money—where it comes from and how to use it.

When he better understood the concept, I let him manage the flow of money in our family. After he graduated from high school in 2006, I handed over the family accounts to him, and he now has his own bank book. He also monitors our family expenses, from water and electricity bills to our monthly parking fees, and he will remind me when it is time to pay the bills. Antonio also examines the reasons for the increase in expenses, controls our expenses, takes care of himself, and does housework: washing, cooking, sweeping the floor. It is very important for Antonio to be able to use money wisely because if I have to leave him one day, he will still be able to spend money wisely.

Today, I can say that I have no worries at all. Antonio can take care of himself, and sometimes me too. I am not worried if I go to heaven tomorrow because Antonio is able to live independently. I always want him to be happy in his family and life, therefore I treat him as an equal. Our relationship between mother and child does not have the feeling of parental superiority. We get along equally and take care of each other.

I wonder if Antonio will consider getting married. He told me that he had favorite classmates when he was in school. As a parent, although you may worry, you cannot deprive your son of the right to like people. Therefore, I thought it was very important to teach him to finish studying, control his emotions, prepare to meet friends or girlfriends, and develop adult relationships.

Macau also has good assisted living facilities for people with disabilities, such as Seng Kong Se and Lar Sao Luis Gonzaga. After I pass away, Antonio can move into one of these homes and his living expenses will be covered by the disability pension from Macao's Social Security Fund, which is around MOP3,740 (around $460 US) per month.

I believe every life is important, and everyone can reach their full potential as long as they work hard and receive the right support. I wanted to provide more opportunities for children and adults with intellectual disabilities, so after I retired from my job at the bank, I started doing more social work.

In addition, for many years, my son Antonio and I received a lot of help from people from every walk of life in society and from many enthusiasts. Antonio had very good training in the special schools. He is now quite independent and able to take care of himself, and for this, we are very grateful. Therefore we would like to pass on this love, utilizing our meager strength and resources to help those children with special needs and their families.

From 2007 onward, through Talent of People Charity Association of Macau in Jiangyong county, Hunan, China, I began to help some high school students who were in poverty. And I came to know that there is no school in Jiangyong County for children with special needs. Many handicapped children have to leave their homes and travel a long distance to Yongzhou City to access special education. I hope, in my lifetime, to contribute a little to establishing a school for special education in Jiangyong County. When I visited Jiangyong county in July 2023, the education bureau there indicated that research is underway with a plan to build a special education school. I am looking forward to the early completion of this special education school in Jiangyong County.

Between 2013 and 2019, I was appointed as the chairlady of the Association of Parents of the People with Intellectual Disabilities of Macau (AFEDMM) where I helped introduce speech and music therapy services at the centers, set up the Sunny Band, and established a musical for people with autism and intellectual disabilities and their parents.

I have also inspired parents of people with intellectual disabilities to set up their own associations, for instance, the Macau Down Syndrome Association and the Association of Parents of the People with Intellectual Disabilities of Yongzhou, Hunan, China. In this way, people with different needs can receive proper support.

In 2016, I worked with other parents to help our children establish the Macau IC2 ("I Can Too") Association. IC2, the only non-government organization that is organized and managed by people with intellectual disabilities and autism based in Macau, is a nonprofit organization that promotes the rights of neurodivergent people. IC2 has conducted workshops, classes, and visits to foster inclusive education, promote cultural exchange, and support individuals with special needs.

After I finished my role as chairlady of AFEDMM in 2019, I became fully involved in the Macau IC2 Association where Antonio had already become the president in 2016. Other members with autism and intellectual disabilities also took up important positions on the board. As parents, we support them and help them operate the association, with things like outreach and financial management. Gradually, we have them take on more responsibilities.

We still have a long way to go, but we are hopeful that they can eventually run it themselves. We want to give them a sense of ownership—empowering them and strengthening their abilities so they can live in society with dignity. Our organization is committed to fighting for the rights and well-being of people with autism and intellectual disabilities, working toward the implementation and application of relevant provisions outlined in the Convention on the Rights of Persons with Disabilities.

To achieve our goals, IC2 has specific targets in mind. We aim to enhance opportunities for participation in community activities, the expression of opinions, and the ability to make decisions. Through various activities, we promote personal growth among individuals with autism and intellectual disabilities. Additionally, we act as a voice, effectively conveying the feelings, needs, and suggestions of these individuals to both the government and society. We emphasize the importance of self-help and mutual support, fostering a spirit of empowerment. Lastly, we strive to raise awareness about the Convention on the Rights of Persons with Disabilities, ensuring that the public recognizes and respects the rights and interests of individuals with autism and intellectual disabilities.

Thanks to the resources from the government that show people with intellectual disabilities and autism can lead a good life, I have supported Antonio in setting up the association, witnessed more and more incoming volunteers and members, organized various activities and courses, and extended our helping hands to more special kids in China.

Macau had been a Portuguese colony since the Ming Dynasty. The Portuguese government was in place until the handover back to China in 1999. After the handover, the government invested a lot of resources in welfare measures, and now after all disabled people are certified, the government will issue disability benefits. There is social security, so there is a certain degree of income security. I believe that the welfare safety net built by the government is relatively complete, and different residential homes can be arranged for those who need them, which is very reassuring for parents.

For more than 30 years, including parenting and social services, my biggest inspiration is the initial transformation from unconscious negativity related to disabilities to the concept of empowering children, which is a valuable experience. Birth, old age, illness, and death are the only way to go through life, and many parents of special children are most worried that they will die earlier than their children, leaving no one to take care of them. Only by allowing children to increase their abilities will parents feel at ease. After all, a parent will grow old, and if she dies, what will happen to her children? Instead of worrying, I recommend that parents of children with disabilities try to help their children live independently while they are alive.

In addition, special children, like ordinary people, will be caught off guard by sudden things. Therefore, I have tried to prepare Antonio, so he will understand that birth, old age, illness, and death are necessary things in life, and when he dies, Antonio will not be too hesitant. I have also arranged for the details related to the "aftermath"— placement of the ashes, the contact person for help in case of an accident, etc.—so Antonio is prepared to deal with the event.

My Recommendations

The most important point is to understand human uniqueness. We need to do our best to understand our children and facilitate their growth and development to be more independent and confident.

My Wish for You

As the mother of an autistic child who is going to turn 40, I feel blessed for the opportunity to understand neurodiversity. My wish is for all to accept and embrace differences and respect each and every human being with compassion and understanding.

Ways to Connect with Me

WeChat - Ruby-b19

Ruby is a pioneer and leader in the disability community in Macau. Here are her most notable positions:

Current:

Parent Council of Macau IC2 Association

Rehabilitation Services Consultant of Macau Coffee and Tea Association (Since 2019)

Board Member of Talent of People Charity Association of Macau (Since 1998)

Previous:

Chairlady of the Executive Board, Association of Parents of the People with Intellectual Disabilities of Macau (2013-2019)

Vice Chairlady of the Executive Board of Association of Parents of the People with Intellectual Disabilities of Macau (2005-2013)

Member of the Commission on Rehabilitation Affairs (2013-2019)

Member of the Advisory Group of the Cross-departmental Study on the 10-year Development Plan for Rehabilitation Services (2016)

Resources

Autism Spectrum Disorder -
https://www.asha.org/public/speech/disorders/autism/

From Linguistic Uncertainty to Professional Resilience

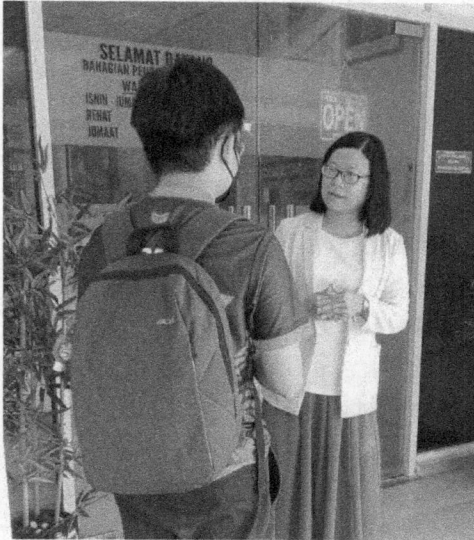

Shin Ying Chu, Ph.D.

朱芯盈

The term "speech-language pathology" was completely foreign to me as I entered the University of Kansas. It remained a novel term as I worked on my psychology degree, as I delved into an introductory course on speech, language, and communication. It was then that I talked to the department chair, Dr. Hugh Catts, to learn more about the field. After finishing the psychology degree, I was excited to continue pursuing a master's degree in speech-language pathology.

During that period, I was hesitant because I didn't feel confident about my English language competency. I thank my clinical supervisors, who demonstrated unwavering support for my language proficiency while conducting clinical work. However, I struggled in report writing and treating patients, particularly when managing patients after having a stroke. I quickly adapted to the working setting, knowing that the program was highly competitive and the intake into the program was minimal. With confidence, diligence, and humility as an Asian student, I collaborated closely with a dedicated group of peers. Together, we tackled the complexities of report writing, dedicated ourselves to rigorous course studies, and engaged wholeheartedly in collaborative group projects. It didn't take long for me to recognize that, despite English not being my native language, I possessed a range of professional skills that could significantly contribute to our team's success.

While pursuing my master's degree, a unique opportunity arose. I was tasked with evaluating a child with a cleft lip and palate (birth defects of the upper lip and roof of the mouth) prior to their cleft revision surgery. Collaborating closely with Dr. Steven Barlow, we embarked on a journey to measure the child's oral pharyngeal pressure—throat contraction pressure—before and after the surgery. This experience was truly remarkable, as it not only provided us with a valuable objective assessment but also left a profound impact on both the child and their family after the revision surgery. As I encountered the child in the clinic parking area, I was pleasantly surprised to hear him pronounce my name, 'Ying,' with perfect accuracy. It was a delightful moment! Later that day, I entered Dr. Barlow's office with a sense of accomplishment, sharing how we had seamlessly bridged research-based evidence and equipment to benefit a real patient. In response, Dr. Barlow smiled and said, "Indeed, that's the impact of science and the role of scientists." This reference to being a scientist left me pondering the true essence of a scientist's responsibilities.

I was raised in a small town in Malaysia and had never been on a flight before I went to the United States. The term "scientist" was unfamiliar to me as well. I am proud to be the first woman in my family to pursue higher education and study overseas. Neither of my parents completed even 12 years of secondary education. Going to the United States was a distant dream I never thought I would achieve. From a young age, I was instilled with values of obedience and respect towards my parents, who had hoped that I would pursue a more traditional career like becoming a lawyer, teacher, or something in that vein. They also hoped that I would study in Malaysia, never thinking I would go overseas to pursue my education. At that time, psychology was an unfamiliar field in my family. However, I chose a different path, one that led me to pursue higher education at a university abroad.

My beloved grandmother and mother have always been a tremendous source of encouragement, fully aware of the challenges that independent work and family life pose for women in Malaysia, particularly for a woman of Chinese heritage, like me. Growing up in a Chinese family in Malaysia, there was a gentle expectation to honor Confucian values, which emphasized family values and loyalty. This often meant conforming to a predetermined path of raising children, maintaining a secure, salaried job to support the family, and adhering to established gender norms rather than pursuing a career that might challenge these expectations.

I was intrigued by the idea of conducting research and asked Dr. Barlow if I should study further for a doctoral degree. Thanks to his support, I obtained a scholarship from the University of Kansas, which supported both my master's and doctoral studies. Thanks to these opportunities, I have learned so much and acquired so many skills. However, I must admit that English continues to be a challenge, particularly when I'm tasked with composing professional journal articles.

This marked the beginning of a difficult journey for me. While I had learned English during my childhood in Malaysia, daily conversations and clinical work didn't pose significant hurdles. Yet, when it came to the intricate art of crafting journal articles, I realized it was an entirely different skill to master. I enrolled in various professional writing courses to develop specific skills on writing, and it was helpful to confront, identify, and correct my grammatical errors. Years later, when I shared this experience with my native English-speaking peers, they too acknowledged that writing journal articles is indeed a unique skill—one that I had erroneously believed was a challenge only encountered by non-native English speakers for many years.

Upon completing my doctoral degree, I had the fortunate opportunity to embark on a new journey in Japan—a novel environment that would challenge me to acquire both a new language and research skills as a postdoctoral researcher. Even though Japan is part of Asia and I'm an Asian, I know nothing about the Japanese language. The culture shock occurred when someone in Japan asked me, 'Why are you doing this? You are married, and why don't you stay at home to raise kids?' Even though both countries are in Asia, the roles and expectations of married and unmarried women within their respective social communities were starkly different. Navigating through documents written in an unfamiliar language added another layer of complexity and consumed a significant amount of my time. In the face of such comments and challenges, I made a conscious decision to disregard the remarks and steadfastly concentrate on my work.

My background of speaking Mandarin, Cantonese, Hokkein, and Bahasa Melayu, really helped me master the Japanese language in a short time. I quickly learned the common daily conversational phrases while meeting with Japanese speakers who stuttered. I thank the lab director, Dr. Mori Koichi, and my associate, Dr. Sakai Naomi, for their patience and for affirming the value of cultural-language differences. The proficiency I had in reading and writing Mandarin proved to be an invaluable asset when I undertook the challenge of learning the Japanese language. This prior knowledge facilitated my mastery of

Japanese in a surprisingly short span of time. I thank my mother, who made the crucial decision to enroll me in Mandarin-speaking schools during my elementary education. Little did I know that this early exposure to one language would significantly impact my ability to learn other languages later. I have never been so proud of my cultural background and of knowing multiple languages.

Knowing that Malaysia lacks speech-language therapists (SLTs), I returned to Malaysia to serve as a senior lecturer at the National University of Malaysia (UKM). For this, I thank Dr. Kartini Ahmad, whom I met at a conference in Taiwan. She suggested that I serve my home country by training future SLTs. My dedication to research, teaching, mentoring, and clinical training has only intensified during my tenure at UKM.

While working with students and delivering services to patients, my multicultural-multilingual background helped me become more culturally competent. Given the increasing globalization and rapid immigration patterns, various factors like race, ethnicity, culture, language, and religion among the individuals we serve can significantly influence how healthcare is received and, consequently, how it should be delivered. Over the last two decades, courses dedicated to multicultural education within speech therapy programs have been developed and textbooks have been published. The American Speech-Language-Hearing Association (ASHA) also has a number of Special Interest Groups (SIGs) with multicultural/global emphases. Still, continuous improvements are needed for cultivating cultural competency among our students.

Even though I was raised in Malaysia with a multilingual-multicultural background, when I started to work with communities outside of my own Chinese ethnicity, I realized how much our beliefs differ. For instance, to promote inclusivity and accessibility of available resources, I needed to prepare the same treatment protocol or instructions for our caregivers in different languages. I currently focus on creating posters to promote the May Better Hearing and Speech Month campaign in Malay, Mandarin, and English to promote awareness of communication disorders and ensure our team communicates effectively with the community we serve. This initiative offers resources that are both physically and culturally accessible to all individuals. By prioritizing inclusivity, we foster a more welcoming and supportive community for individuals of all backgrounds and abilities.

In summary, based on my personal experience, the following are some of the important components that assist me as a multicultural competence academician. When reflecting on my background, I realize that I have adopted the five elements of the process of developing cultural competence, as proposed by Campinha-Bacote: cultural awareness, cultural knowledge, cultural skill, cultural encounters, and cultural desire.

1. *Cultural awareness.* One must understand his/her cultural life experience, explore the implications of their background culture for health care, and be aware of their biases or prejudices towards other cultures. From my experience, a willingness to explore different cultures could help my clients

realize their own ethnocentricity.

2. *Cultural knowledge.* As a speech therapist, I strongly recommend not to be afraid to ask and understand other cultures and to gain knowledge regarding other ethnic groups. Acquiring such cultural knowledge can greatly assist in effectively caring for patients from backgrounds different from our own.

3. *Cultural skills.* Speech therapists are expected to communicate with individuals of different cultures, conduct assessments, and continue to learn how to conduct culturally based assessments. We must remind ourselves of the importance of verbal and non-verbal (body) language, eye contact, and the power of silence, which can hold distinct meanings across various cultures.

4. *Cultural encounters.* With globalization, speech therapists must equip themselves to serve disabled communities across the world. Developing cultural sensitivity occurs through exposure to and engagement with diversity within cultural groups, which is crucial in preventing stereotypes about specific communities. This will also prevent stereotyping towards a certain community. An effective approach to increasing cultural exposure is to engage in internships or fellowships within culturally diverse outpatient clinics, as this can significantly enhance one's cultural sensitivity.

5. *Cultural desires.* This is a personal motivation to become culturally aware and knowledgeable, to

seek cultural encounters, and to become more skillful. Personal experience of exposure to various cultures could help enhance the desires and practice the knowledge one's learned in the clinical settings.

My Recommendations

In my capacity as a multilingual speech therapist and educator, I offer these personal suggestions to you as you continue your journey of serving and gaining deeper insights into various communities. This lifelong journey fosters curiosity, passion, resilience, and a profound appreciation for making a meaningful impact on society.

Below are the lessons I have learned:

- I've come to understand the importance of following my passion and embracing challenges. When confronted with obstacles I can't immediately overcome, I've learned to trust my instincts, go with the flow, and find enlightenment in life.

- I've recognized that learning is an ongoing, lifelong journey. The pursuit of knowledge fuels my curiosity, deepens my wisdom, diminishes my prejudices, and encourages me to persevere in my continuous research efforts, all with the aim of making a positive impact on the society I serve.

- I've come to appreciate the value of sharing as an act of giving. Inspired by my mentors, I've realized my willingness to share knowledge and skills with my peers, students, and the community, fostering collective growth within our field of speech therapy.

- I firmly believe that each failure represents a unique learning opportunity, bringing us one step closer to achieving our ultimate goals.

- I've learned to cherish and express gratitude for every individual I've met, each community project I've been involved in, and every research endeavor I've undertaken. These experiences collectively contribute to my personal growth and resilience.

- I've acquired the ability to embrace the cultural distinctiveness of each individual and to respect the choices made by others.

I hold a deep passion for educating future clinicians and extending community services to those in need. These aspects of my career and life bring me immense joy and satisfaction. It's at times like these that I truly understand the wisdom in the old Chinese saying, "It is more blessed to give than to receive" (施比受更有福). I am profoundly grateful for the incredible mentors, peers, friends, and collaborators who consistently encourage me to embrace challenges, offer their assistance when needed, and provide unwavering support. Their contributions have played a pivotal role in various aspects of my professional growth, including publications, grants, teaching, and personal development.

I thank my parents, who always embrace our culture and have been very proud of teaching us Chinese culture ever since I was young. This strong cultural background and foundation and sense of identity have empowered me to serve as a global citizen. I share these insights for those who are open to, contemplating, or already engaged with the various communities with disabilities:

1. Show respect for other cultures and be attentive to their beliefs and needs.

2. Always try to understand other people's cultures. You will be surprised by how willing people are to share their cultural traditions and beliefs with you.

3. Prioritize inclusivity and accessibility when working within diverse cultural and disabled communities. These are vital principles to ensure the effectiveness of your efforts.

Ways to Connect with Me

Email: chushinying@ukm.edu.my

Dr. Chu is an associate professor in the Faculty of Health Sciences at the National University of Malaysia. Her research areas focus mainly on understanding speech motor control and the quantification of speech motor performance in both normal and disordered populations. This research has been focused on developing assessment tools for patients with Parkinson's disease and stuttering. Most recently, her specific interests are concentrated on examining the social participation of patients with communication disorders and on developing evidence-based practices among Asia's allied health professionals.

Finding the Light Inside with the Child and the Families

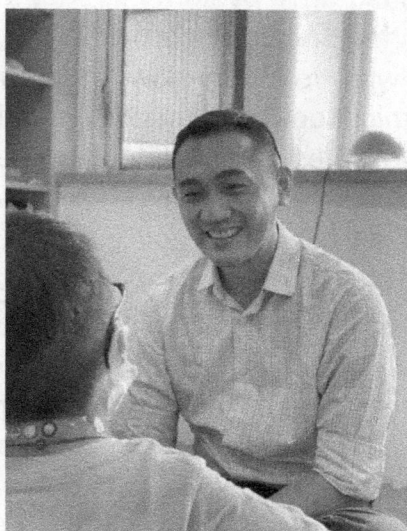

Tony Ching-Hsien Chang, M.S.

張敬賢

In the early summer of 2001, at the age of 24, I had just graduated from the university's psychology department and completed my mandatory military service. Soon after, I began my first full-time job. I joined as a team member of the Early Intervention Assessment Center in a medical center in Taoyuan County. My role was to assist the doctors in the Department of Pediatric Rehabilitation gathering information and chief complaints from the families of children with suspected developmental delays before their appointments.

Because the Taiwanese government implemented a national health insurance system in 1995, it allows citizens to pay monthly health insurance premiums based on their income levels with relatively low fees, making various necessary examinations and treatment affordable. Early intervention assessment and intervention services are also covered by the insurance system. Parents are encouraged to participate in assessments and interventions; however, there are typically long wait times for appointments and high patient caseloads, and staff availability is limited. Most physicians tend to provide a preliminary diagnosis to anxious parents onsite, in an attempt to ensure qualification for services. This is typically a more general diagnosis (e.g., suspected developmental delay, suspected ASD). However, due to the challenges of obtaining ongoing intervention, the initial diagnosis is never fully verified, is often incorrect, and ultimately misrepresents the child's actual needs.

Additionally, popular intervention facilities also have a long queue from several weeks to months. To manage the waiting list, intervention session durations are shortened, with most common sessions in Taiwan often lasting 30 minutes per week, provided either one-on-one or with one therapist for two or more children. The busy schedules lead therapists to experience continuous fatigue and go through the pressure in a limited time for either evaluation or intervention. Over time, the cumulative fatigue and numbness in response to therapy are not always the results they expected.

My workspace at the time was in the waiting room next to the doctor's consulting room. I remembered the tense and anxious appearance of most parents who entered the waiting room for the first time. In the beginning, most of the parents began to share, talking in a hurried and cautious tone, however after I spent 15 to 30 minutes with the family and child, some of their nervous emotions began to ease, and the parents typically left with more relaxed expressions, while the children looked back with big smiles and cheerful waves.

Experiencing these small exchanges in expressions of gratitude, I felt that I had finally started my journey into the human services industry after leaving the university. Although I played a relatively minor role in the early intervention work teams, it seemed like my work was genuinely delivering some help for families of children with developmental needs. My role provided them with clearer information and allowed them to face the subsequent processes with less confusion. During the two years I worked there, my colleagues and I interacted with over two thousand new families with early intervention needs. Day by day, I felt that I was doing reasonably well as a young professional and was satisfied with my role on the team.

Around the spring of 2003, the Severe Acute Respiratory Syndrome (SARS) epidemic in northern Taiwan was winding down, quarantine restrictions were eased, and people began returning to their previous lives.[1] One day a mother arrived carrying her four-year-old son wrapped against her chest. During the interview, I learned they had previously undergone basic examinations and assessments at other hospitals, and her son had been diagnosed with congenital brain development abnormalities, along with ventriculomegaly (a condition where the brain's ventricles, or fluid-filled spaces, are larger than usual) and macrocephaly (having a larger head size than typical, often due to an enlarged brain or other factors), generalized muscle hypotonia (a medical term for decreased muscle tone, making muscles appear floppy or feel unusually soft and making it harder to move or hold up the body), global delay in all development areas, and inability to use meaningful speech for communication. He expressed wants and needs through crying and emotions rather than verbal or gestural means. Though the mother wore an N95 mask, her distress was evident from her expressions.

She explained that this was her first child, and the family hadn't noticed the development issues of the boy until his first birthday. Since then, she had been shuttling between various local hospitals and clinics on her own, as her husband was fully occupied with work and unable to give more time to accompany her. In addition, her mother-in-law blamed her for the child's condition and believed

---

[1] MLA Citation: "Severe Acute Respiratory Syndrome (SARS) | Virus, Disease, Symptoms, & Facts." Encyclopedia Britannica, https://www.britannica.com/science/SARS. Accessed 4 October 2023.

that it was due to defects in the mother's family genes that their first-born grandchild turned out this way.

In traditional Taiwanese culture, it was common for at least one child in a family to live with the husband's parents after marriage to maintain the concept of "continuing the family line." Traditional values emphasize descendants, particularly male offspring, should carry on the family name, inherit any property, and uphold the family reputation through generations, so it's expected that they be healthy and robust to shoulder the responsibilities. While modern society has become more accepting of different family compositions, this practice was still prevalent in Taiwanese households over two decades ago. Discussions on this topic typically revolved around issues of gender equality and marital relationships. However, for families of children with special needs, especially when a male child was diagnosed with developmental delays, the challenges that typically arise from communal living went beyond traditional family dynamics, created internal strife, and became a catalyst for endless arguments. Most mothers of children with developmental issues faced significant blame and emotional stress from the elders in the family. They carried the burden of self-blame, loneliness, high pressure, helplessness, and various related psychological health issues.

Meanwhile, most fathers either couldn't face the situation or were unable to defy their own parents. Within traditional Chinese virtues, filial piety, or "being good to one's parents," is highly emphasized. Under the banner of filial piety, fathers often refrain from opposing the opinions and decisions of their parents. This dynamic might result in internal family conflicts arising from doubts about the child's mother inheriting genetic defects, as well as differences in parenting perspectives across generations. The father's role is often passive or silent, maintaining a sense of absence. Furthermore, regarding taking the child outside for therapy, the elderly in the family often refrain from support based on the traditional notion of "family shames must not be spread abroad" or "not airing dirty laundry." They might even prevent such actions.

By the end of the intake interview, I knew the mother was suffering. Her son hadn't been able to respond to any screening materials and activities, and the room was full of the boy's crying sounds. As I retrieved several parent questionnaires from the file cabinet, intending to hand them to the mother to take home, she abruptly inquired, "What are these? I don't want to fill out more of these things," before I could explain their purpose. Without pausing for my response, she went on, "My child should be starting elementary school given his age, but he still struggles to understand or complete many tasks. I came here to seek immediate help for my son." She continued with a hint of despair, "My husband couldn't help me, the previous doctors couldn't help me," then pushing the questionnaires back towards me, asserted, "and YOU CAN'T HELP ME, EITHER!" With that, she stood up and stormed out, leaving my colleagues and me stunned.

I remembered the feelings and thoughts echoing in my head following this event. I felt sorry for her and her son, and I found myself inadequate and powerless as I realized there was nothing I could do to support her. I was ashamed and angry at my earlier feelings of satisfaction and accomplishment. It was the first time I deeply understood that early intervention should not only focus on the data and numbers on paper, or the child's noticeable performance and development progress but also on the family members who raise and support the child. For these families, the professional team members can offer more support and resources, and I could personally do a lot more than just finding ways to serve beyond "doing reasonably well."

Because of that mother's emotional story, I felt awakened and began to think, "I want to do more than sitting behind the desk." Not long after, I left that job and enrolled in the graduate school of the Department of Speech and Hearing Sciences and Disorders at the National Taipei University of Nursing and Health Sciences.

After entering the clinical practice as a speech-language pathologist, my main service involved children with various communication needs. To adapt to different work demands, I went from hospital therapy room to mountain aboriginal tribes, from the high-end urban residences to courtyards of iron sand factories. I started my journey by shedding the white coat and moving out of my comfort zone of the air-conditioned rooms, and my immature work attitude began to change.

From working with these children with special needs, I've learned that a child's smile while completing a story-expanded activity in a bright, tidy room is similar to another child's delighted smile after writing down his own name with muddy hands. Both smiles represent the same level of confidence and joy. Through the interaction between the children and their parents, I observed while one child constantly asked questions to her mother with curiosity, and the mother patiently answered each time. Another child kept showing his mother a fascinating toy he discovered during the game. The mother warmly embraced her child, expressing their love and connection through non-verbal communication. The interaction between parents and the children involves not just verbal but various other possibilities to convey warmth.

They helped me understand that love takes many different forms and achieving goals involves many different paths. There is no one-size-fits-all intervention strategy in this world. It helps me accompany children and parents to find the best path for them, like their own light in the darkness, ensuring that every step is more solid than the previous one, helping parents lead their children forward steadily. I'm grateful for all this. It's made me no longer the bewildered and powerless young person in the office. Now, I can use my professional skills to accompany and influence children with special needs and their families towards a more confident direction. Through this journey, I've found the confidence to continue progressing and working harder.

My Recommendations

Based on all my experiences, ongoing education, and guidance, I would like to share the following personal recommendations with you as you contemplate the Asia-Pacific ethnic cultural disability community.

1. Accumulating multidimensional professional learning experiences is essential.

When we encounter cases of special needs individuals, instead of viewing a client solely through the lens of a disability or impairment, it is vital to perceive the individual as a "whole person" with diverse needs. In the Asia-Pacific region, within the realm of special needs professional work, the comprehensive involvement of the service recipients may not always be possible. This may be due to the variation in policies among different countries and regions, disparities in medical resources within each area, and the diverse levels of support and resources available within individual families. Professionals who can provide direct services to clients need to learn to comprehend a wide array of different fields of knowledge. Flexibility in approaches is crucial for coping with various special needs. Thereby it enables the development of intervention programs which is best suited to the needs of service users through collaborative discussion and planning.

2. Stand by the service recipients' side to accompany and grow together.

In the cultural context of the Asia-Pacific region, medical professionals are often perceived as possessing absolute authority. As frontline specialists in special needs, when engaging with service users and their families, professionals need to understand the importance of standing beside them with empathy before commencing professional interventions. Engaging families as collaborative partners in discussions to develop intervention plan goals fosters a tailored and cooperative relationship in accordance with the family's structure and needs. Considering the diverse development needs across various stages of the service users, intervention objectives and strategies need timely adjustments. Based on the needs, professionals need to continuously assimilate knowledge relevant to different life stages and engage in ongoing discussions with families. Utilizing a dynamic adaptive approach is essential for developing the most suitable intervention plans for the service users and their families.

3. Understand one's limitations and respect all aspects of different cultures.

   Human services professionals not only require expertise in their field but also the recognition of their role's limitations. For instance, we cannot provide all answers or replace the role of the client's family in fulfilling any family function. Our role can participate in specific stages of the service recipient's life journey, but we cannot make decisions for the entire life of our client. While we provide professional services based on our role, we cannot fulfill all the needs of the service recipient on an individual basis. We can act as a coach for the family, guiding them progressively with our professional skills, discussing the adjustments after practical application, and ultimately leading to empowering family members.

In Asia-Pacific region societies, as opposed to Western countries, there is a strong inclination toward collectivism. It often leads to an environment that values consensus and group harmony, and potentially overlooks the real cultural diversity present in individuals' daily lives. Factors such as language, religion, residential area, and upbringing contribute to diverse cultural attributes and individual characteristics. Respecting their culture and avoiding imposing the professional's cultural viewpoint on the service recipient facilitates consensus in intervention strategies that better align with their real-life contexts.

My Wish for You

If you and your family are special needs service users, please remember that you and your family are unique and irreplaceable in the world of special needs family members. By allowing them to participate in home activities while they progress and grow, they gain valuable life experiences, language demonstrations, and emotional communication, which cannot be substituted by the intervention of the most exceptional professionals. While caring for your dear family members, remember to pause and take care of yourself. When you are filled with strength, you can accompany them for a longer journey.

If you are just starting or are currently on a journey to understand human services professionals' work, you may have completed or are about to complete numerous professional courses. Congratulations on getting closer to the ideal job every day. During your learning journey, keep an open mind. Besides challenging professional subjects, it's crucial to improve knowledge in the area of the humanities. In the middle of the hard work of learning, take time to listen to your inner voice. Try to explore and understand better the reasons behind your inclination to become a helping professional. Self-examination and reflection will help you find the strength to keep moving forward.

If you are contributing to innovative changes in supporting special needs service work, it's an honor to have you as a partner in the effort. I believe that through your professional growth and accumulation, you've gained valuable experiences. We should continue to learn and not forget to appreciate the various forms that have given us the strength to grow along the way and keep learning the wisdom of life from the special needs community we care about. Even if our individual strength is small, remember that near you or on the other side of the world, there are partners with the same goal. Together, let's strive to make high-quality professional service work shine in the corners of different cultures.

Ways to Connect with Me

Email: tonychang.cch@gmail.com

Facebook: @tony.chang.1656

My name is Tony Chang, and I am a speech language pathologist from Taipei, Taiwan. My professional interests include communication and symbolic behavior development in children with special needs. I have been practicing in a center of speech and language intervention program in a university setting, and I have worked with families of children with special needs facing difficult challenges in each stage of their children's growth process. Through my work I have learned so much and am very grateful to share my stories with some of the children and families here.

The Sign Language Teacher Who Never Gives Up

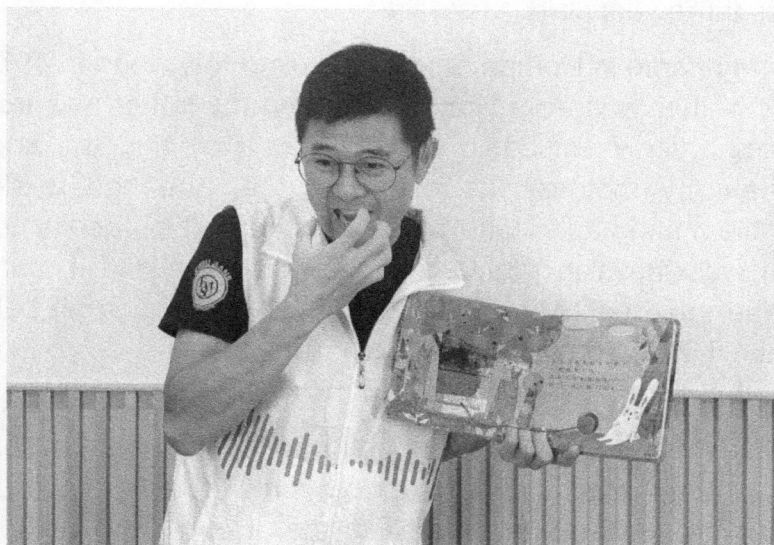

Un, Ho Man; Homan

源浩民

When did you leave home?

I still have a vivid memory of that day. The sun was shining brightly, and I was still unsteady on my feet. My mother hugged me tightly, her expression full of anxiety. She was saying something to me, but it sounded like gibberish. We got on a big boat that took us to another land. There, we met two women who looked like my mother. I found out later that we had moved to Hong Kong, a place I had been to before, but this time it was different because I said goodbye to my parents and started living with my grandma and my aunt. It was the year 1982, and I was three years old.

My name is Homan, and I came into this world in 1979. My mother was from Hong Kong, and my father was from Macau. They settled in Macau after they tied the knot. When my mother was expecting me, she had a skin problem and had to take some Chinese herbs. I don't know if it was the skin problem or the herbs that did it, but it made me Deaf. My mother thought I was a normal baby when I was born, but after three months, the doctor told her that I had no hearing and that it was very bad.

You might know about Hong Kong, but maybe you don't know about Macau. They are both small cities in the south of China. Macau is even smaller than Hong Kong, with an area of less than 30 square kilometers. Macau only has 700,000 people living there even now. There were no schools for Deaf people in Macau back then. My mother wanted me to have a good education, so she sent me to a school for Deaf people in Hong Kong.

Do you think that going to a school for Deaf people meant that I could finish my education easily, like anyone else, and then join society, get a good job, and become who I am now? The answer is "no way!" For some background information, I need to explain the outcome of the "Milan Conference" (the first international conference of deaf educators), which was held in Milan, Italy, in 1880.

Out of 164 delegates from seven identified countries represented, only one participant was deaf: James Denison from the United States. As a result of this conference, eight resolutions were passed supporting oralism (oral education) over manual education (sign language). The people attending the conference thought that sign language would make it hard for Deaf people to learn and fit in with normal society.

As a result of this conference, many Deaf schools, including mine in Hong Kong, did not allow sign language to be the main way of teaching for all subjects. They preferred that Deaf people try to be oral to communicate with the hearing population. However, for Deaf people, our first challenge is hearing, and this makes it difficult to learn and produce oral language. Our ears are there, but they don't work well. That was before electronic implants were common. I always had to bring a device to help me hear things. It was like a big power bank that I kept in a bag on my chest. It had two wires that went to earphones in my ears.

Although I had been learning how to speak Cantonese since I was little, I still struggled to speak. When I went to Macau to see my mom on holidays, she would take me to different places and teach me words by orally producing them on the back of my hand. That way, I could feel how they sounded coming from her lips and mouth and say them along with her. My parents and relatives would always try to teach me new things, like playing word games at restaurants and showing me Chinese characters on menus. They would also help me with talking and reading skills. That's how I learned to know food pictures and words. The first food word I learned was "fish balls"—I love them! But once I ordered bitter melon by mistake instead; I've hated it ever since.

In first grade, I only knew a few words and had trouble expressing myself. When I got to secondary school, the language became harder for me. The sentences were longer and the words were more complex. I was not able to "hear" what the teachers were saying. I finished high school and wanted to study business practice, but it was not easy. The classes were large, and the teachers spoke fast. I had to get extra help from them after school to barely pass the course.

You might be wondering, "If school didn't help you much, why did you choose to become a teacher?" Well, the truth is, I learned a lot in school, and those lessons became the foundation of my teaching philosophy. My school for the Deaf emphasized oral communication, requiring students to speak in class and outside of it. But my friends and I weren't very good at speaking, so during breaks, we secretly learned Hong Kong Sign Language (HKSL) from our senior peers. If the teachers caught us signing, they would stop us, but chatting and sharing life stories were too important to us. So we communicated in sign language privately. Sign languages were developed by Deaf people for the purpose of communication. It is a spatial language using gestures, finger spelling, and writing to express communicative intent. Sign languages are now recognized as languages and are taught in a majority of deaf schools, although not worldwide.

Since I couldn't hear, the second thing I learned was the importance of "seeing." When I didn't understand something written, I focused on the pictures and tried to understand the text from them. When I didn't know a word, I asked friends or family or looked it up in a dictionary. I taught myself how to read and write better by reading comic books, magazines, and newspapers.

Although I worked hard in school, as a disabled person, my job search wasn't easy. After graduating from high school, I tried working as a clerk and a chef at a pizza shop, but those jobs didn't last long and didn't give me much satisfaction. My father was a professional water and electricity line repairman, so I worked with him. Although I couldn't hear, learning how to repair water and electricity systems was no problem for me. In fact, I was able to repair them in my own home!

By chance, my Deaf friend in Macau brought me to volunteer at the Macau Deaf Association and learn Macau Sign Language (MacSL). Even though it was 2003, I found out that Deaf children in Macau were still like me when I was young—they were only allowed to learn oral language. Worse still, there were no Deaf schools in Macau, and children couldn't chat with their senior peers in sign language!

Then fate intervened like playing Monopoly—Chance or Community Chest cards appeared. My old classmates in Hong Kong told me that the Chinese University of Hong Kong offered sign language courses and invited me to study with them and eventually become a teacher. I hesitated because my water and electricity line repair skills were already mature enough for me to take over my father's business. Also, I had no experience teaching children and was worried that I wouldn't be able to learn how to be a teacher.

I chose the Chance card: I made a choice to pursue my dreams and challenge destiny. Luckily, I was accepted into the program, passed the required courses, and graduated from the Chinese University of Hong Kong in 2016. Eventually, I became a Deaf teacher at the Macau Deaf Association's Education Center for Children with Hearing Problems.

Do you think Deaf teachers are the same as hearing teachers? I can tell you for sure, they're not! The traditional way of teaching sign language is to follow the Chinese grammar rules for each word—this is called "Signed Chinese." But I am Deaf myself, and I know that sign language should be learned naturally. So I use daily conversations and games to teach children natural sign language. If children don't understand something, I use facial expressions and gestures to show them sign language so they can also have fun while learning.

Besides teaching, I also help parents and children communicate better—fixing "common communication problems"—because I was once a child too and am able to understand their feelings of frustration and confusion. Parents write me letters in Chinese about the issues they face when raising their children, and I use sign language to teach children how to respect their parents, solve problems, and also use real-life family situations to teach them more sign language.

Since becoming a sign language teacher, I continue to expand my knowledge by reading a lot of books and writing reports; I sometimes even look for information on the internet. This makes me realize how important reading and writing are for learning. So I include these components in my courses too.

I don't think that being Deaf automatically makes someone a good teacher for other Deaf people. I have seen that Deaf children are very diverse in their abilities and personalities—some are more intelligent than others; some are shyer; some progress slowly; some have other challenges—so I keep learning new things to improve my teaching skills.

Helen Keller once said, "The only thing worse than being blind is having sight but no vision."

I moved away from home when I was three years old and stayed in Hong Kong for 20 years before coming back. As a Deaf person, I am paving the way for a brighter future where Deaf children can stay at home longer, learn sooner, and come back home with achievements more than ever before.

My Recommendations

1. Society should provide equal access to education and work for Deaf people so they can also participate and contribute to the common good.

2. Deaf people should not doubt their own abilities. Everyone has different gifts. As the proverb says, "Every cloud has a silver lining." I wish that every Deaf person can discover their own strengths and

use them to the fullest.

3. When you are capable, assist others without expecting anything in return. Others may benefit from your assistance and transform their lives.

Ways to Connect with Me

Email: unhoman@gmail.com ; homan.un@mda.org.mo

YouTube: https://www.youtube.com/@KidsCanSignMacau

Interests: Bowling, surfing the internet, and raising cats

Un Ho Man is a Deaf teacher who works at an education center for children with hearing impairments, affiliated with the Macau Deaf Association. He graduated from a Deaf school in Hong Kong and returned to Macau, where he initially worked as a plumber. In 2016, he seized the opportunity to train as a sign language Deaf teacher and pursue his passion for helping Deaf and hard-of-hearing children. He is 44 years old and has a wealth of experience and knowledge to share.

The following people assisted Un Ho Man to write his chapter:

- Mother: Sham Siu Lan（沈少蘭）

- Sister: Un Man Yee（源敏儀）

- Colleague: Leong Chao Man (梁秋雯）

Ho Man's mother shared many stories about his youth, and he is thankful that with her help, he was able to recall how he learned to communicate. His sister is a teacher and provided editing for his chapter. His colleague provided a translation from written Chinese to written English.

Struggling to be Heard

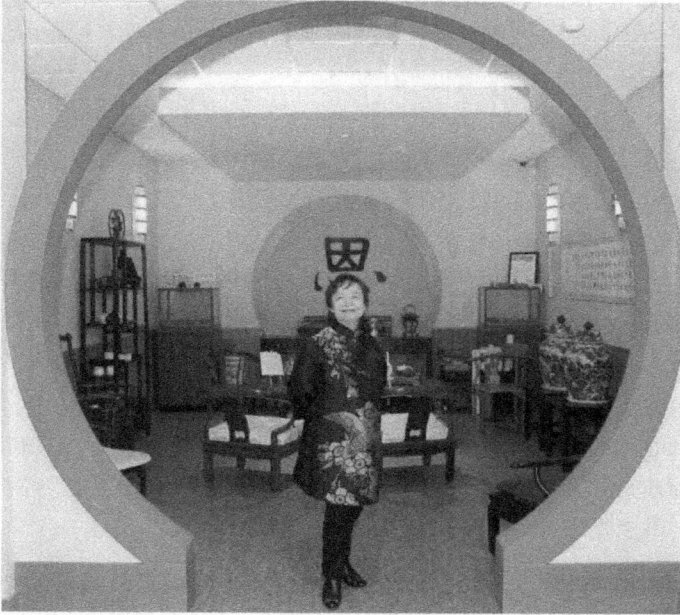

Li-Rong Lilly Cheng, Ph.D., CCC-SLP

劉麗容

Many decades ago, I was considering the study of speech pathology, so I made an appointment to see the dean of the College of Communication at Michigan State University to get his advice. He encouraged and advised me, instead, to study audiology because I would not be required to use so much English. I took his advice and applied to the department to pursue audiology. I did exceptionally well in my coursework.

While I was taking courses in speech pathology and audiology, a faculty member with an Asian background encouraged me to go into speech-language pathology. She said the field needed people like me with a solid bilingual background. As an international student, I was hesitant because I didn't feel confident about my English language competency. But she encouraged me, and with her strong support, I finished all the required courses with excellent grades. She was correct; my bilingual background was an asset, not a deficit, even though I did not realize it then. Many years later, I was given the honor of being named an outstanding alumnus. So, I thank her for having confidence in me and affirming the value of bilingualism.

As part of the requirements for graduation, I needed to complete 375 hours of clinical contact. I worked with clients in several settings to gain all of the required hours. Although I did very well in my coursework, I was concerned about my clinical assignments. I was worried because I needed more exposure to American culture, looked different, and spoke with a foreign accent. As a speech-language pathology student, I felt inadequate to work with native speakers of English. I felt my foreignness was a problem.

My first assignment in 1972 was at a school for the deaf, and my first client was a deaf and blind student. In a way, I was relieved and thought this was a good assignment. I felt a sense of relief because the person was blind and could not see my yellow skin, and he was deaf and could not hear my foreign accent. I worked hard to figure out how to communicate with him. Helen Keller was my inspiration, and I felt empowered by reading about her and integrated using the sense of touch to work with this client. My on-site supervisor was empathetic and helped me with this very challenging client. The department chair who created the assignment wanted me to experience success, and I thanked him for his foresight and careful consideration.

My second assignment was to work in a state hospital. My classmates warned me that this was a terrible assignment, and I soon found out they were correct. I had to travel for an hour in the severe winter to get to the state hospital. I was told to walk with my back toward the wall and watch out for anyone who might approach me. I was given clients who were nonverbal and violent. All the doors were locked, and one of my clients was a huge blind fellow who got angry very easily. One day, he threw an oversized chair at me, and luckily, I was not injured. The environment was hostile and dangerous, and I had almost no supervision. It was a very challenging and trying time. Even so, my Chinese background of swallowing bitterness sustained me, and I finished my assignment without missing one day.

My next assignment was in a school, and I had to work with students with articulation problems. My supervisor was not happy with my pronunciation of the /th/ phonemes. I understood her concerns and worked very hard to improve my pronunciation. My Confucian influence made it acceptable to listen to her comments because she was my teacher/supervisor. In those days, there was no accent reduction program. Later, many departments offered accent reduction programs, which evolved into accent modification programs. I do not personally advocate this type of program. I believe communication enhancement is a much better way to approach this challenge. To enhance cross-cultural communication, one needs to be competent not only in language forms and content but also in pragmatics.

Over the last four decades, I have learned the importance of mentoring and having mentors. The first time I encountered the word "mentor," I did not know what it meant. I learned that this word was the name of a Greek person the emperor had trusted to teach his son. My first mentor, Professor May Chin, suggested that I study speech-language pathology. As a second-generation Chinese American, she did not have the opportunity to continue speaking her mother tongue Cantonese. Once she entered kindergarten, her family wanted her to speak fluent English, and she soon lost the ability to speak Cantonese. She became monolingual, and later in life, she discovered how important it is to be bilingual and bicultural. She encouraged me to study speech-language pathology because she thought that I had the linguistic capability to speak Mandarin and Cantonese and could serve the Chinese-speaking population. Studying speech-language pathology was a massive challenge for me because, in those days, most of the students were native speakers of English. I was the only one in my class whose mother tongue was not English. On occasion, my professors and fellow students could not understand me, and I could not understand them.

I also want to share my experience with one phenomenal mentor, Dr. Katharine Butler, who served twice as the president of the American Speech Language and Hearing Association and twice as the president of the IALP (formerly known as the International Association of Logopedics and Phoniatrics) the International Association of Communication Sciences and Disorders.

I remember our first encounter at a California Speech and Hearing Association annual convention in 1985 where I was giving a talk about bilingualism. After the conference, she invited me to write a book based on my knowledge about the Asian populations. I was unprepared to embark on a writing journey; I struggled to write short papers because my writing style was circular, and I was slowly learning the linear style of writing. She empowered me and affirmed me. Years later, I was elected to serve as the president of the International Association of Communication Sciences and Disorders, and I think of her all the time.

The book that Dr. Butler encouraged me to write took two and a half years, and after three years of work, the book was finally in print in 1987. The publisher sent me the first copy of the cover to keep. I shared it with my department chair, who placed this page on our bulletin board. I had to teach a class early that evening, and when I returned to the department, I noticed that the book cover was completely covered with swastika signs. I froze and could not believe my eyes. The only thing I could do was remove it from the bulletin board. This hurt me deeply. I felt numb, humiliated, speechless, and shocked. The trauma was unspeakable, and the pain was unbearable.

I did not share this experience with anyone for at least a year. I could not understand why anyone would do that to deface the cover of my book. Did I mention that the title of my book is *Assessing Asian Language Performance*?

After years of living in the United States, I began to realize I needed to become more socially aware and culturally adapted to my environment. I began my quest to understand the socially acceptable patterns of behaviors and interactions in America. I used the Review, Interview, Observe, Trial (RIOT) approach, initially designed to be used in educational contexts as a framework for gathering information to evaluate underlying causes of academic or behavioral problems exhibited by students.

For the "R" (review) component, I read American history and biographies of famous people. I also read the books that American high school and college students usually read. In fact, there is some cultural knowledge that most Americans organically obtain throughout childhood that helps them assimilate in mainstream US society, in addition to common literary pieces such as Jack and Jill and *Tom Sawyer*, by Mark Twain. I needed to know what this was and so I focused on explicit cultural knowledge, the apparent aspects of culture that can be learned by asking questions or observing. I had to do a deep dive to acquire linguistic competence. Much of what I had to learn to be competent linguistically involved implicit culture. For example, there are straightforward questions that can be asked socially and questions that should not be asked. There are issues regarding what is appropriate and what is not. These are the elements that must be studied and understood thoroughly. Otherwise, it is tough to move on. Without these foundational elements, I believed advancing as a well-rounded professional would be challenging.

I employed the "I" (interview) component to gain knowledge of the implicit culture. I began to ask pertinent questions about socially and culturally acceptable behaviors. I found many variations of what is appropriate, depending on the context and persons involved. A simple example would be asking about someone's age in China, which is very common. The reason for asking the question about age is to place oneself in the social order of seniority. In contrast, age is considered something personal in the United States. Consequently, this question should not be asked because it would be considered inappropriate and rude. In addition, there is also the implication of possible age discrimination. This led me to dig deeper into the implicit cultural elements. I still have a long way to go as this is a lifelong journey.

The next step was the "O" component, given that the implicit culture is hidden and cannot be easily observed or detected. As mentioned earlier, what is implied in American culture is the idea of individualism and the idea of independence. On the contrary, growing up on the island of Taiwan which practices interdependent and collectivist culture differs from the individualistic way of thinking. This is where the hidden agenda or curriculum concept comes into play. Where can one acquire knowledge about behaviors deemed socially acceptable?

The most important approach is based on observation within the targeted culture. An American child would know what a typical picnic looks like. A child growing up in China will have a very different concept of a picnic.

"T" stands for trial and error, defined by learning and understanding differences (i.e., What is appropriate or inappropriate). Newcomers/learners will certainly make missteps or errors while learning a new culture. It is essential not to be too easily discouraged as this is part of learning a new culture. It is necessary to react to these errors using humor (e.g., I'm learning slowly). One may also share information about the social rules in their own culture, as this will help others understand that their behavior was not an error but was based on a different cultural upbringing.

I have certainly learned many lessons from my years as an academic. These invaluable experiences have inspired me to continue improving my understanding of my multiple identities, being female, Asian, Chinese, American, Cantonese, a speech-language pathologist, mother, wife, and professor. I have often been asked for advice on surviving and thriving academically.

Below are the lessons learned:

- I learned to excel in what I do and continue to pursue and engage in the pursuit of wisdom, knowledge, and skills. I try to be the best I can be in my expertise. In addition, I try to find my passion or the fire inside me. My passion drives me to continue improving and achieving my goals.

- I learned not to be afraid of challenges and take risks. I gain confidence from failures, biases, and discrimination. Risks are part of life; taking calculated risks may lead to unexpected outcomes.
- I learned to ensure I have mentors and a circle of supporters. I heed the advice from my mentors and reflect on their comments and guidance. In addition, I serve as a mentor and do as much as I can to help those who need mentoring.
- I learned to find inspirational role models. These are people that can inspire me even in my darkest moments. My role models include Mother Theresa, Wole Soyinka, Nelson Mandela, Walter Munk, Paulo Friere, Helen Keller, and Ruth Bader Ginsburg.
- I learned to believe in continuous improvement (CI). I improve my multilinguistic, multicultural, and cross-social competencies. The goal of attaining competence is always a work in progress and will always continue because I firmly believe in the value of gaining competence as a global citizen.
- I learned to use the RIOT method (record review, interview, observation, and test). It is critical in many aspects of my academic career and beyond. The more reviews, interviews, and observations I can do, the better prepared I am for testing my theories.
- I learned to understand the importance of "give and get. " When I am willing to give, I get a lot. So, we must plan on sharing more, whether in service in our profession or volunteering for community activities.

- I learned to stay hungry and stay foolish. As Steve Jobs said, "Stay hungry, and stay foolish."
- I learned to stay curious. Your curiosity quotient will also drive your success. When you do not understand why certain things are done in a certain way, ask questions and do a deep dive. The discovery process may be challenging and sobering, but it is the journey we must travel to attain our goals.
- I learned that being bilingual/multilingual is an asset, not a deficit. Being multicultural is a shared reality for many, and advocating for this form is crucial.

Being different is part of my DNA. I have found strengths in all the journeys I have taken and all the encounters I have experienced. What has sustained me is the comfort in continuous lifelong learning and in knowing that there is always light at the end of the tunnel. I fully understand that being different goes beyond being marginalized, oppressed, and disenfranchised. I sincerely appreciate my mentors who asked me to never give up, never despair, help when I can, and care more than I should. My multicultural experiences also have given me strength, resilience, and humility. They have also contributed to my teachings, publications, and interactions with individuals across the globe. There is always a story behind each person; as stated in the following poem, I am WHOLE. I have traversed my *nepantla* (a term used by Nahuatl to mean "in the middle of it" or "middle") and I have integrated my multiple selves.

Struggling to be Heard

Li-Rong Lilly Cheng

I am a child of the Chinese diaspora, born at a crossroads.

I am a Chinese-American,

A product of the city of Shanghai I have never known.

An immigrant and the daughter of Cantonese,

I speak Cantonese with love, the language of Dim Sum and Chinatown.

I speak English with passion; it's the tongue of my consciousness,

It is my crystal, my tool, my craft.

I am from Taiwan island grown, and Taiwanese is my dream,

Ripples from my tongue rest in my heart,

I am from Pacific Asia, a stranger from a different shore, deeply rooted in history.

I am from California; I love the city of San Diego.

I am Asian, Asia is in me, but I cannot return.

I am Chinese, China lives in me, but there's no way back.

I am Taiwanese. Taiwan remembers me, but I have no home there.

I am new. History made my hyphenated existence. I was born at the crossroads, and I am whole.

My embraced multiculturalism matters and is central to my journey.

My Wish for You

My overall wish for the readers is that we are connected as human beings and that we must learn to listen to each other and care for one another.

My Recommendations

I share these personal recommendations with you as you consider your contributions to the community of people of Asian Pacific Islander culture with disabilities.

- Cultures are not static but dynamic—learn to adopt, adapt, and create your own culture based on your value system
- Cultivate empathy and listening skills
- Develop your skills in observation and dialoguing guided by respect
- Respect diversity and neurodiversity

My Community

Listen to my interview on the Xceptional Leaders Podcast with Mai Ling Chan:

https://bit.ly/li-rongcheng

Ways to Connect with Me

Email: Lcheng@sdsu.edu

Dr. Li-Rong Lilly Cheng is the founding director of the Chinese Cultural Center and was a professor in the School of Speech, Language, and Hearing Sciences at San Diego

State University. She is the past chair of the American Speech-Language Hearing Association (ASHA) Multicultural Issues Board and the past president of the International Association of Communication Sciences and Disorders (IALP). She served on the editorial board of several major professional journals. She has published numerous articles and books. She is a frequent keynote speaker on the topic of neurodiversity, cultural diversity, East meets West, language learning, and language disorders. She holds visiting professorships in multiple universities. Her honors and awards included ASHA Honors, ASHA Fellow, ASHA Multicultural Contributions, and Diversity Award from the California Speech & Hearing Association. Dr. Cheng has also served as a consultant for *Sesame Street* and Tiffany and Company.

Final Thoughts

Drawing from the profound insights and shared wisdom of 15 disability leaders of Asian Pacific Islander (API) heritage, this anthology culminates in a rich tapestry of narratives that transcend the boundaries of culture and personal experience. As each chapter unfolds, the depth of truth, vulnerability, and interconnectedness reveals itself, offering a glimpse into the souls of those who lead with resilience and grace.

The stories within these pages are more than just accounts of personal triumphs and trials; they are invitations to peer into the heart of what it means to navigate the complexities of disability within the nuanced framework of API culture. The authors have generously opened the doors to their lives, sharing pivotal moments that have not only shaped their paths but also the landscape of disability leadership.

As you journey through these concluding thoughts, reflect on the echoes of your experiences within these shared stories. The vulnerability laid bare in these pages is a testament to the courage it takes to raise silent voices and lead with authenticity in a world that often overlooks the quiet strength of diversity.

In this final chapter, we extend an invitation to you: to learn from these leaders, find solace in their shared experiences, and take up the mantle of advocacy with renewed vigor. Let their journeys inspire you to embrace your own path with courage and to contribute your voice to the ever-growing chorus calling for change.

Here are some steps to consider as you move forward:

1. Connect with the authors through the resources provided, and engage with the broader community they represent.

2. Find inspiration in the resilience and dedication evident in each story, and let it fuel your commitment to making a difference.

3. Reflect on the cultural insights offered, and consider how you can apply this understanding to foster greater inclusivity within your sphere of influence.

4. This anthology is not just a conclusion but a beginning—a call to action for each reader to become a beacon of change and a leader in their own right. Let the wisdom contained here guide you as you step into a world where every voice, including those once silent, is heard and valued.

We offer our sincere thanks for the time you've shared with us, delving into the depths of our experiences. It is our collective hope that these stories have sparked a light within you, illuminating a path to a life and career that is as rewarding as it is impactful. May the ripples you cast forth extend far beyond your immediate circles, enriching lives and strengthening your communities. We are here to support your journey toward becoming a light of exceptional leadership in your community. Let our stories be the wind beneath your wings, propelling you toward a future where every voice, sign, and gesture is heard and celebrated.

www.ingramcontent.com/pod-product-compliance
Lightning Source LLC
Chambersburg PA
CBHW022051020426
42335CB00012B/641